S0-EIG-108

CONTENTS

     1. Aging

     2. Death and Dying

     3. Ethics in Health Care and Scientific Research
         (General)

     4. Euthanasia and the Right to Refuse Medical Care

     5. Genetics

     6. Health Care Professional/Patient Relationship

     7. Human Experimentation and Informed Consent

     8. The Mentally and Physically Handicapped

     9. Patient's Rights and Confidentiality

     10. Prenatal Diagnosis and Intervention

     11. Serious Illness and Pain Management

     12. Other

HUMAN VALUES IN MEDICINE AND HEALTH CARE

Audio-Visual Resources

COMPILED BY NADYA SHMAVONIAN

Printed in the United States of America by
Vail-Ballou Press, Inc., Binghamton, N.Y.

Library of Congress catalogue card number: 82–13394
International standard book number: 0–300–02975–6

10   9   8   7   6   5   4   3   2   1

Introduction

This is a select listing of audio-visual resources which examine human values questions in medicine. The listing includes films, videocassettes, audiocassettes, and slide and filmstrip presentations. A topical index is provided which allows the reader to locate items by subject matter, and to choose a desired format, i.e., video, audio, or panel discussion and lecture.

The first section is composed of an alphabetical listing of visual and audio programs. Each entry includes a technical description of the item, the names of both producer and distributor, and a brief summary of the content. The descriptions are compiled from responses to a national survey of human values programs in medical schools, from comments of informed medical educators, and from summaries provided by producers.

Panel discussion and lecture series are in a separate appendix. In general, these series were produced in academic settings for initial use in teaching situations. Each videotape in the appendix examines a specific issue, and the titles of these tapes are usually self-explanatory.

Following the appendix is the topical index, a comprehensive listing of titles under twelve general subject headings which are then subdivided according to format. While many of the entries included cover issues in several different areas, each item is listed only once under the major topic being considered.

Finally, the full names, addresses, and telephone numbers of distributors for all programs in this listing are provided.

It is perhaps interesting to note that despite the large selection of audio-visual resources available, the national survey revealed that only a small number of films and tapes were used widely among medical schools. They are: "The Anatomy Lesson," "Dying," "Hospital," "Please Let Me Die," "Who Should Survive?," and "Whose Life Is It Anyway?"

A project of this kind can never be considered complete; new releases will quickly outdate the listing, and some valuable existing productions have no doubt been overlooked. Nonetheless, it is hoped that this listing will provide a useful guide to audio-visual material currently available for use by persons who are exploring human values questions in medicine and health care.

Recommendations from members of the Society for Health and Human Values and from other individuals working in human values programs were useful in finding audio-visual material that was suitable for this listing. Catalogs of educational media distributors were also helpful in providing information. Reviews and summaries from the following organizations were valuable: The National Library of Medicine, Concern for Dying, Filmakers Library, Lowengard & Brotherhood, National Public Radio, Time-Life Video, and the Trainex Health Care Library. Special thanks are extended to Sandra Bertman, Associate Professor, Humanities in Medicine, University of Massachusetts Medical Center, for her audio-visual reviews in Death Education, and for her help in all phases of this project.

Nadya Shmavonian

HUMAN VALUES IN MEDICINE AND HEALTH CARE:

AUDIO-VISUAL RESOURCES

AN ADOLESCENT COPES WITH CANCER (1979, 3/4" videocassette, 27 min, col)
    Production: St. Louis University Medical Center; Alice Dean Kitchen
    Distribution: St. Louis University Medical Center; $95 for purchase;
      $25 for rental

An interview with an adolescent who is dying of cancer. His feelings
about imminent death and response to treatment are expressed.

AGING: EXPLORING THE MYTHS (1979, audiocassette, 59 min)
    Production: National Public Radio
    Distribution: National Public Radio; $7 for purchase

Professionals and lay persons explore stereotyping the elderly, their
growing political power, and how other countries treat their older population. Dr. George Maddox, Director of the Center for the Study of Aging
and Human Development, Duke University; Elias Cohen, Project Director, Law,
Aging and Long-term Care, Public Interest Law Center, Philadelphia; Robert
Butler, Director, National Institute on Aging; and Maggie Kuhn of the Grey
Panthers discuss losing mastery, retirement, societal expectations, sex,
family roles, and work potential.

THE ANATOMY LESSON (16mm film, 30 min, col)
    Production: Margaret Bole
    Distribution: Embassy of the Netherlands; free loan

A filmed ballet of Rembrandt's 1632 painting, "The Anatomy Lesson of Professor Tulp." The dance was choreographed by Glen Tetley, and performed
by members of the Nederlands Danstheater, with music by Marcel Landowsky.

AND WE WERE SAD, REMEMBER? (1978, 16mm film, 3/4" videocassette, 29 min, col)
    Production: Department of Health, Education and Welfare, Office of Librar-
      ies and Learning Resources, Office of the Deputy Commissioner for School
      Systems
    Distribution: National Audiovisual Center; $250 for 16mm purchase; $65
      for 3/4" purchase; $25 for 16mm rental.

Children's reactions to death and family interaction concerning funerals
are examined.

ARE YOU DOING THIS FOR ME, DOCTOR, OR AM I DOING IT FOR YOU? (1975, 16mm film,
    3/4" or 1/2" videocassette, 52 min, col)
    Production: BBC; Peter Jones, Peter Goodchild
    Distribution: Films, Inc.; $700 for 16mm purchase; $350 for 3/4" or 1/2"
      purchase; $75 for 16mm or 3/4" rental

This program raises questions about ethical standards in medical experimentation, such as whether fully informed consent is a realistic possibility.
The ethics of experimentation with prisoners, the mentally retarded, institutionalized persons, and minors are discussed in this program. The doctor-
patient relationship is analyzed in the context of problems in providing
informed consent.

ATTITUDES TOWARD DEATH AND DYING (1974, 3/4" videocassette, 30 min, col)
   Production: Jefferson Cable Corporation, Channel 10, Charlottesville;
   Thomas H. Hunter, William Smith
   Distribution: University of Virginia, School of Medicine; $24 for out-of-
   state rental; $19 for Virginia rental

   A tape of the program, "People, Places, and Things," covering such topics
   as the following: attitude toward death, brain death, terminal care,
   passive euthanasia, truth-telling, tissue donors, decision-making, economics, and physicians' duties.

BECKY: THE VALUE OF A LIFE (1977, 16mm, 24 min, col)
   Production: Joseph P. Kennedy, Jr. Foundation
   Distribution: Lowengard & Brotherhood; $185 for purchase; $25 for rental

   Ethical problems of informed consent are presented. Becky Braznell, a
   hydrocephalic, was institutionalized as a young girl and given a short life-
   expectancy. She outlived these expectations, but the quality of her life in
   the institution was poor. When her parents learned of another child in need
   of a transplant for renal failure, they volunteered Becky as a donor, hoping
   to give her life new meaning. The ethical questions surrounding this case are
   discussed.

BEHAVIOR CONTROL
   (see series: "Hard Choices" - Part 4)

BEING PART OF IT ALL (1981, 16mm film, 3/4" videocassette, 24 min, col)
   Production: Richard Burman
   Distribution: Filmakers Library; $450 for 16mm purchase; $400 for 3/4"
   purchase: $45 for 16mm rental

   This film introduces a Canadian couple, Gary and Barbara, who are mentally
   handicapped. Although they both met and spent most of their lives in an
   institution, they decided to marry and establish themselves independently.
   Their family and community are seen as important to this adjustment, and the
   film encourages the viability of such a marriage, provided these support
   systems are present.

BERTHA (1973, 16mm film, 35 min, col)
   Production: Joseph P. Kennedy, Jr. Foundation
   Distribution: Lowengard & Brotherhood; $230 for 16mm purchase; $25 for
   16mm rental

   Bertha, born into a poor family of ten children, has been labeled mentally
   retarded. She spent her childhood in foster homes, and was a constant
   truant before leaving school after seventh grade, unable to read. At fifteen
   she was sent to a diagnostic institution, where professionals recommended

the implantation of an intra-uterine device. Her parents were not con-
sulted because she was a ward of state. The ethical issues raised by
this case are discussed in the film.

BIOETHICS IN GENETIC COUNSELING (1978, series in 3 parts, slide and audio-
cassette, col)
Production: Medical College of Pennsylvania, Teaching Program in Human
Values in Medicine; Garrett E. Bergman, John H. Sorenson
Distribution: Council on Education and Science; Pennsylvania Medical
Society; $5 for single program rental

Part 1. BIOETHICS IN GENETIC COUNSELING: DOWN'S SYNDROME/AMNIOCENTESIS
AND ABORTION (54 slides, 25 min, guide)

The interplay of ethical and clinical aspects in the case of a thirty-eight
year-old primagravida is examined. Faced with the high risk of bearing
a child with Down's Syndrome, this couple chooses amniocentesis, knowing
that it is only a diagnostic tool, not a treatment. They opt for an
abortion upon positive diagnosis. Alternatives to these choices are
considered.

Part 2. BIOETHICS IN GENETIC COUNSELING: TAY SACHS DISEASE AND GENETIC
SCREENING (40 slides, 20 min, guide)

Part Two of the "Genetic Counseling" series considers the criteria which
need to be met for the identification of carrier status to be ethically
sound. The importance of confidentiality is stressed. How such screening
can provide guidance for couples identified as carriers is considered.
Special emphasis is placed upon alternative patterns of relationship in
doctor-patient counseling.

Part 3. BIOETHICS IN GENETIC COUNSELING: PKU AND CYSTIC FIBROSIS:
STERILIZATION AND ARTIFICIAL INSEMINATION (57 slides, 25 min, guide)

The impact of two genetic diseases which are similar in that they are
treatable but not capable of being diagnosed in utero is considered.
The two couples in this presentation are at high risk because they have
each had a child with one of these genetic diseases. One couple decides
to "play the odds" and have another child of their own even though the
risk of occurrence of genetic defect is high. The other couple chooses
sterilization to birth of another genetically-diseased child.

BIOETHICS IN NURSING PRACTICE (1981, series in 5 parts, filmstrip and audio-
cassette, or slide and audiocassette, col)
Production: Robert J. Brady Co.
Distribution: Robert J. Brady Co.; $450 for filmstrip series purchase;

$585 for slide series purchase; $100 for filmstrip single program purchase; $130 for slide single program purchase

This series presents bioethical problems in nursing practice.

Part 1. BIOETHICS IN NURSING PRACTICE: ACCOUNTABILITY IN NURSING PRACTICE

Part 2. BIOETHICS IN NURSING PRACTICE: PATIENT ADVOCACY IN NURSING PRACTICE

Part 3. BIOETHICS IN NURSING PRACTICE: HUMAN RIGHTS IN NURSING PRACTICE

Part 4. BIOETHICS IN NURSING PRACTICE: WHO LIVES, WHO DIES, AND WHO DECIDES

Part 5. BIOETHICS IN NURSING PRACTICE: THE MORAL VALUE IN HEALTH CARE

BIO-ETHICS: WHO'S IN CHARGE HERE? (1978, audiocassette, 59 min)
Production: National Public Radio
Distribution: National Public Radio; $7 for purchase

Dr. Bruce Hilton, Director of the National Center for Bio-Ethics, discusses some of the dilemmas which have arisen as a result of scientific advances. He focuses on the process of amniocentesis as a diagnostic process. He also discusses mood-altering drugs, the Living Will, and the Karen Quinlan case.

BOY OR GIRL: SHOULD THE CHOICE BE OURS?
(see series: "Hard Choices" - Part 1)

C.J.
(see series: "People You'd Like to Know" - Part 1)

CAN'T IT BE ANYONE ELSE? (1980, 16mm film, 3/4" videocassette, 32 min and 54 min versions, col)
Production: John Korty, Bill Couturie
Distribution: Pyramid Film and Video; $695 for purchase, $75 for rental (long version, 16mm or 3/4"); $450 for purchase, $60 for rental (short version, 16mm or 3/4")

Three children (ages ten to twelve) with leukemia are the focus of this program. The ways in which these children have confronted their diseases are observed, as well as the feelings of their families.

CARE OF DYING CHILDREN (1978, audiocassette, 52 min)
Production: National Public Radio
Distribution: National Public Radio; $7 for purchase

Dr. Bill Bartholomew, Professor of Pediatrics at the University of Texas, gives an address on the "Care of the Child Dying of Cancer." He discusses the importance of discovering a child's sense of self; a child's lack of understanding of personal and physical time; the stages in a child's understanding of death; the role and impact on doctors and nurses; and dying at home or in the hospital. Audience discussion follows.

THE CHALLENGES OF AGING: CHANGE AND LOSS (1976, filmstrip and audiocassette, 3/4" or 1/2" videocassette, 15 min, col)
    Production: Trainex Corporation
    Distribution: The Trainex Health Care Library; $90 for filmstrip purchase; $140 for 3/4" or 1/2" purchase; $13 for filmstrip rental (must order minimum of 5 programs); $55 for 3/4" or 1/2" rental

    Problems of change and loss in aging are examined in this program. Reactions to the following are recorded: change in kinship role, loss of family, change in social role, loss of social contacts, change in environment and loss of familiar surroundings. These changes and losses are seen to affect the individual's needs for emotional warmth, belonging, independence, dignity and self-esteem.

CHILLYSMITH FARM (1981, 16mm film, 3/4" videocassette, 55 min, col)
    Production: Mark Jury, Dan Jury
    Distribution: Filmakers Library; $750 for 16mm purchase; $650 for 3/4" purchase; $75 for 16mm rental

    This film is a ten-year record of one family's experience with death and aging. Based on the book, Gramps, it portrays the shift from the family's dependence on Gramps to Gramps' dependence on the family as his death approaches.

A CONVERSATION WITH A WIDOW (1977, 3/4" videocassette, 30 min, col)
    Production: University of Arizona, Health Sciences Center
    Distribution: University of Arizona, College of Medicine; $145 for purchase; $25 for rental

    A dialogue between a social worker and a woman in her early sixties whose husband was a cancer victim is presented. The woman is open and articulate in describing the stages of grief she and her husband experienced. The program provides insight into the life and emotions of a person suffering the loss of a mate after twenty-six years of marriage.

COPING WITH CANCER (1981, 3/4", 1/2", or 1/4" videocassette, 24 min, col)
    Production: Kaiser/Permanente Medical Center
    Distribution: Professional Research; $295 for purchase; $50 for rental

The feelings and experiences of individuals coping with cancer are examined. The program presents new ideas for counseling cancer patients and their families.

COPING WITH SERIOUS ILLNESS (1980, series in 6 parts, 16mm film, 3/4" or 1/2" videocassette, each program 30 min, col and b&w, guide)
  Production: Time-Life Video
  Distribution: Time-Life Video; $2,500 for 16mm series purchase; $1,100 for 3/4" or 1/2" series purchase; $300 for series rental; $600 for 16mm single program purchase; $225 for 3/4" or 1/2" single program purchase; $60 for single program rental

Experts in medicine, psychology, patients' rights, consumer rights, law, and finance examine Joan Robinson's struggle with terminal illness.

Part 1. PAIN

Different approaches to coping with both pain and the fear of pain are shown in this program. The effects of pain upon personality are discussed, as are different types of pain, and methods for its treatment.

Part 2. DOCTOR/PATIENT RELATIONSHIPS

The relationship between Joan Robinson and her doctor and other medical personnel is examined. Experts discuss the important factors in choosing a doctor, and the special bond that develops between dying patients and their doctors. Clergypersons and nurses also discuss their relationships with dying patients.

Part 3. SEXUALITY

Physicians and other experts examine the issue of the sexual and loving needs of seriously ill patients.

Part 4. RELATIONSHIPS

Experts examine methods for coping with the changes in relationships that result from the diagnosis of serious illness.

Part 5. FINANCES/INSURANCE

The financial aspects of serious illness are examined in this program. The ways in which the Robinsons handled their bureaucratic and financial problems are studied. Insurance experts discuss selecting proper coverage, and a lawyer discusses wills and estate planning.

Part 6. FACING DEATH

Joan and Eric Robinson are shown as they face the reality that Joan will die. Different families' responses to the diagnosis of terminal illness are discussed, such as whether to die at home, in a hospital, or in a hospice. Physicians, psychiatrists, clergy, and others join in the discussion.

DAVID (1980, 16mm film, 3/4" videocassette, 28 min, col)
    Production: Canadian Broadcasting Corporation
    Distribution: Filmakers Library; $425 for 16mm purchase; $375 for 3/4"
    purchase; $45 for 16mm rental

    David McFarlane, a sixteen-year-old with Down's Syndrome, is shown in this
    program. He is an articulate, athletic and poised young man who has just
    acted the lead role in a television drama about mongolism. He enjoyed his
    work, for which he won an international award. He discusses his life, and
    the problems his handicap has caused. His family is introduced, and their
    support for David is examined.

DAVY IS ENTITLED
    (see series: "The Family and Its Relationship to the Developmentally
    Disabled: Legal, Ethical and Moral Issues" - Part 2)

DEAD BIRDS (1963, 16mm film, 3/4" videocassette, 83 min, also available in
    three 28 min parts, col)
    Production: Robert Gardner
    Distribution: McGraw-Hill for purchase; CRM/McGraw-Hill Films for rental;
    $895 for 16mm series purchase; $695 for 3/4" series purchase; $395 for
    16mm single program purchase; $295 for 3/4" single program purchase;
    $63 for 16mm series rental

    New Guinea intertribal warfare and death are shown in this film. Mourning
    and grief rituals are examined also.

DEATH (1969, 16mm film, 43 min, b&w)
    Production: Arthur Barron; Evelyn Barron
    Distribution: Filmakers Library; $400 for purchase; $40 for rental

    Albro Pearsall, a fifty-two-year-old man dying of cancer in a New York
    hospital is portrayed. The film records the hospital routine and the
    responses of staff, family, and patient to terminal illness. Questions
    are raised concerning communication with dying patients, and psychological
    responses of both patient and staff to terminal illness. Pearsall's
    personal reflections upon his life are thought-provoking.

DEATH AND DYING (Mid-1970s, audiocassette, 24 min)
    Production: Trainex Corporation
    Distribution: The Trainex Health Care Library; $9.95 for purchase

Dr. Elisabeth Kubler-Ross discusses death and dying in our society. Dr. Kubler-Ross' theory of the five stages of dying includes: denial, anger, bargaining, grief, and acceptance.

DEATH AND DYING
    (see series: "Hard Choices" - Part 5)

DEATH AND THE DOCTOR
    (see series: "Working with Death" - Part 1)

DEATH BY REQUEST (1976, 16mm film, 25 min, col)
    Production: Michael Ryan
    Distribution: Concern for Dying; $300 for purchase; $25 for rental

    This is the story of seventy-eight-year-old Meg Murray, a widow with multiple
    sclerosis living alone in the English countryside. She has been ill with MS
    for forty years, but is afraid that when she declines to the point of wanting
    death, she will be so disabled that suicide will be physically impossible.
    She wishes to repeal the English law which makes assisted suicide a criminal
    act. She believes that all people should have the right to decide for them-
    selves the time of death, and to request help if needed. Barbara McNulty, a
    nurse psychotherapist, discusses problems of this request. She argues that
    if all dying patients had the right to choose when to die, many would feel
    compelled to end their lives prematurely in order to avoid becoming a burden
    to their families.

DEATH OF A GANDY DANCER (1977, 16mm film, 3/4", 1/2", or 1/4" videocassette,
    26 min, col)
    Production: Learning Corporation of America; Michael Blum
    Distribution: Learning Corporation of America; $425 for 16mm purchase;
      $325 for 3/4", 1/2", or 1/4" purchase; $40 for 16mm rental

    A fictional film about a family trying to cope with a dying member. Ben
    Matthews, a retired "gandy dancer" (railroad man), is dying of cancer.
    Initially, his daughter and her husband try to keep their knowledge of
    his imminent death from Ben, but as his pain worsens he realizes that he
    is going to die. He asks that his 10 year old grandson, Josh, be included
    in family discussions of his death, because he feels there is nothing shame-
    ful about death to hide from the boy.

THE DEATH OF A NEWBORN (1976, 16mm film, 3/4", 1/2" or 1/4" videocassette,
    32 min, col)
    Production: Case Western Reserve University, Health Sciences Communi-
      cation center
    Distribution: Polymorph Films; $450 for 16mm, 3/4", 1/2" or 1/4" purchase;
      $45 for 16mm rental

This program depicts the trauma and grieving process resulting from the death of a newborn. A case history is recorded in interviews with the parents of a dying infant. The parents' need for support during this stressful period is articulated.

DECISION FOR THE 80s: GENETIC ENGINEERING (1980, audiocassette, 59 min)
    Production: National Public Radio
    Distribution: National Public Radio; $7 for purchase

Dr. James Dewey Watson, Nobel Laureate in Bio-Chemistry, and Representative George Brown (D., CA), of the House Committee on Science and Technology, discuss the problems and rewards of genetic engineering. They consider the role of the Congress and of the Supreme Court in applying controls in this area, and speculate on commercial exploitation of scientific discoveries. Participants in the audience ask about birth defects and patient self-determination.

DEE
    (see series: "People You'd Like to Know" - Part 2)

DETOUR (1977, 16mm film, 3/4", 1/2", or 1/4" videocassette, 13 min, col)
    Production: Caroline Mouris
    Distribution: Phoenix Films; $240 for 16mm purchase; $175 for 3/4", 1/2",
      or 1/4" purchase; $25 for 16mm rental

This program is filmed from the perspective of an eighty-three-year-old woman dying of cancer. Catherine Hamilton is dying in a large hospital, and the viewer experiences the constant activity which surrounds the patient. While Catherine Hamilton tries to die in peace, the hospital staff struggles to keep her alive.

DIANA
    (see series: "People You'd Like to Know" - Part 3)

DIANA: ONE FAMILY'S EXPERIENCE
    (see series: "The Family and Its Relationship to the Developmentally
    Disabled: Legal, Ethical, and Moral Issues" - Part 7)

A DIGNIFIED EXIT (1980, 16mm film, 3/4" videocassette, 26 min, col)
    Production: Granada Television International
    Distribution: Filmakers Library; $450 for 16mm purchase; $400 for
      3/4" purchase; $45 for 16mm rental

A film produced in response to the London Exit Society's attempt to publish a manual on how to end one's life painlessly. The manual was not published, because it is illegal in Britain to aid someone in committing suicide. Three

individuals who because of their personal experience with illness and death
are proponents of the right to choose to die on one's own terms, discuss
their beliefs. In opposition to these individuals, two doctors who work in
the care and support of the terminally ill, speak of advances in pain control.
Many ethical questions are raised in this documentary.

DOCTOR, I WANT ...
    (see series: "Hard Choices" - Part 6)

THE DOCTOR-PATIENT RELATIONSHIP (1977, 3/4" videocassette, 25 min, col)
    Production: Creighton University School of Medicine
    Distribution: Learning Resources Center, Bio-Information Center,
      Creighton University; $11.50 for rental

    A lecture discussion of the ethics involved in the doctor-patient relation-
    ship.

DOCTOR-PATIENT RELATIONSHIPS
    (see series: "Coping with Serious Illness" - Part 2)

DONNIE (1977, 3/4" videocassette, 20 min, col)
    Production: RMS Productions
    Distribution: Learning Resources Center, Bio-Information Center, Creighton
      University; $11.50 for rental

    The question of who is responsible for a child born with multiple physical
    impairments is raised.

A DOSE OF REALITY (1977, 16mm film, 3/4" videocassette, 16 min, col)
    Production: Suzanne St. Pierre, CBS
    Distribution: Carousel (CBS) Films, Inc.; $325 for 16mm or 3/4" purchase;
      apply for rental information

    Joy Ufema, a "death and dying" nurse, is profiled in this segment from a
    60 Minutes program. Joy argues for dying patients' need to participate in
    treatment plans and decisions. Families she has worked with are interviewed
    in this program, as well as the director of her hospital.

DREAMS SO REAL: THREE MEN'S STORIES (1981, 16mm film, 3/4" videocassette,
    28 min, col)
    Production: Oren Rudavsky, with the N. G. Nord Centers, Lorain, Ohio
    Distribution: Filmakers Library; $475 for 16mm purchase; $425 for 3/4"
      purchase; $45 for 16mm rental

A personal view into the needs of mental patients attempting to make the transition back into the community. Three outpatients from a community mental health center are presented through their words and through animated films they created. The dreams and realities of their lives are recorded in this program.

DREAMSPEAKER (1977, 16mm film, 3/4" videocassette, 75 min, col)
    Production: Canadian Broadcasting Corporation
    Distribution: Filmakers Library; $995 for 16mm purchase; $700 for
        3/4" purchase; $100 for 16mm rental

A cross-cultural look at attitudes toward death; a Canadian boy is contrasted with an older Indian shaman, Dreamspeaker. The boy is troubled, and has run away from society. The two befriend one another, but the boy is found by authorities and taken back to his community. Both Dreamspeaker and the boy choose to end their lives once they are separated, but for different reasons, and with starkly contrasting attitudes.

DYING (1976, 16mm film, 3/4" videocassette, 97 min, also available in 3 parts, col)
    Production: WGBH; Michael Roemer
    Distribution: King Features Entertainment, Inc.; $800 for 16mm purchase;
        $400 for 3/4" purchase; $150 for 16mm rental

Four families' experiences with terminal illness and their personal resources of strength are examined.

THE DYING PATIENT
    (see series: "Working with Death" - Part 2)

EDUARDO THE HEALER (1978, 16mm film, 54 min, col)
    Production: Richard Cowan; Douglas Sharon
    Distribution: Pennsylvania State University, Audio Visual Services;
        $667 for purchase; $28 for rental

This documentary portrays Eduardo Calderon, a fisherman, sculptor, and shaman who uses incantations, psychology, and hallucinogenic drugs to heal villagers in Peru. It offers a cross-cultural contrast to modern technology. (Spanish dialogue with English subtitles.)

ELEGY (1981, 16mm, 7 min, col)
    Production: Debra Zalkind, Jay Cohen
    Distribution: Filmakers Library; $250 for purchase; $30 for rental

A dance program, choreographed and danced by Debra Zalkind. The program offers a visual interpretation of understanding the loss of a loved one.

ELIZABETH
    (see series: "People You'd Like to Know" - Part 4)

ETHICAL AND MORAL DILEMMAS (1975, audiocassette, 58 min)
    Production: Association for Clinical Pastoral Education, E. J. Meyer
     Memorial Hospital, and the Department of Psychiatry, School of
     Medicine, State University of New York at Buffalo
    Distribution: Communications in Learning; $12.50 for purchase

    Ethical and religious questions raised in medicine are discussed.

THE ETHICAL CHALLENGE
    (see series: "Science and Society" - Part 3)

ETHICAL-LEGAL ASPECTS OF NURSING PRACTICE (1974, 16mm film, 3/4"
    cassette, 30 min, col)
    Production: American Journal of Nursing Co., Educational Services Division
    Distribution: American Journal of Nursing Co. (New York) for purchase;
     American Journal of Nursing Co., Videotape Library (Chicago) for rental;
     $395 for 16mm purchase; $265 for 3/4" purchase; $30 for 3/4" rental

    Two issues are confronted in this program, both of which are illustrated
    with examples. In discussing death with dignity, the options open to the
    nurse in caring for a dying patient and his or her family are indicated.
    The right to refuse treatment, the Living Will, and family rights are
    covered. The discussion of human subjects in research includes options
    open to the nurse and the responsibilities of the nurse as an investigator.

ETHICS AND MEDICINE (1977, 3/4" videocassette, 23 min, col)
    Production: Creighton University School of Medicine
    Distribution: Learning Resources Center, Bio-Information Center,
     Creighton University; $11.50 for rental

    A discussion of the relationship of ethics to medicine. Terminology is
    defined.

THE ETHICS OF FETAL EXPERIMENTATION (1975, audiocassette, 51 min)
    Production: Pacifica Tape Library; Paul Ramsey
    Distribution: Pacifica Tape Library; $12 for purchase

    This program emphasizes the need to evaluate the ethical problems involved
    in fetal experimentation more seriously.

THE ETHICS OF GENETIC CONTROL
(see series: "Science and Society" - Part 1)

ETHICS OF MEDICINE AND PSYCHIATRY (1977, 3/4" videocassette, 29 min, col)
Production: American Humanist Association, at WNED-TV, Buffalo, New York
Distribution: American Humanist Association; $175 for purchase; $39 for
rental

A number of ethical issues in medicine and psychiatry are presented. Included
are: doctor-patient relationship, government funding, health insurance, human
rights, passive euthanasia, malpractice, commitment of the mentally ill, and
mental disorders.

ETHICS OF SCIENTIFIC RESEARCH (1977, 3/4" videocassette, 28 min, col)
Production: American Humanist Association, at WNED-TV, Buffalo, New York
Distribution: American Humanist Association; $175 for purchase; $39 for
rental

A number of ethical issues involved in scientific research are presented.
Included are: technology, genetics, intelligence, recombinant DNA, risk,
human experimentation, public opinion, social control, social responsibility,
social values, government funding.

ETHICS, VALUES AND HEALTH CARE (1980, 8 filmstrips and audiocassettes, 20 min
each, col, guide)
Production: Concept Media
Distribution: Concept Media; $98 for single program purchase

These eight filmstrip/audiocassette units provide an overview of major
bioethical issues currently facing the nursing profession. In various
complex clinical situations, nurses are faced with realistic dilemmas,
conflicts and confrontations which are resolved through values clarification, patient advocacy and accountability. A discussion session allotted
for viewers precedes commentary on the situation by nursing educators in
bioethics. Controversial issues, such as abortion, euthanasia, and nurse-
physician relationships are addressed inconclusively, enabling the viewer
to make an individual assessment.

The individual eight filmstrips are listed as follows: The Nature of
Ethical Problems, Values Clarification, A Patient's Bill of Rights, Insti-
tutional Policies, Patient Autonomy, Nurse/Physician Relationship, Nursing
Obligations, Concerning Death.

EUTHANASIA (1978, audiocassette, 59 min)
Production: National Public Radio
Distribution: National Public Radio; $7 for purchase

Yale Kamisar, a Professor at the University of Michigan Law School, speaks on the topic, "A Life No Longer Worth Living: Are We Deciding the Issue Without Facing It?" Drawing upon the Karen Quinlan case, Professor Kamisar first distinguishes between active and passive euthanasia, then argues that active euthanasia is acceptable in selected cases. His principal criterion is the inability of the brain to function at a minimal level.

THE FACES OF A-WING
(see series: "To Age Is Human" - Part 2)

FACING DEATH
(see series: "Coping with Serious Illness" - Part 6)

THE FAMILY
(see series: "Working with Death" - Part 3)

THE FAMILY AND ITS RELATIONSHIP TO THE DEVELOPMENTALLY DISABLED: LEGAL, ETHICAL, AND MORAL ISSUES (1979, series in 7 parts, 3/4" videocassette)
Production: Central Conference of University Training Program in Developmental Disabilities
Distribution: Michigan Media; $25 for single program rental

Part 1. GROUP HOME LIVING: A MOVEMENT TOWARD INDEPENDENCE? (29 min, b&w)

The advantages and disadvantages of establishing substitute family structures in group homes are examined.

Part 2. DAVY IS ENTITLED (58 min, col)

Examines the parental role in helping Davy, a "Triage Level III" child, move from referral to classroom programming.

Part 3. PARENT POWER: A LOOK AT THE PARENT INFORMATION CENTER OF CINCINNATI (32 min, b&w)

The Parent Information Center of Cincinnati (PIC) is presented in this program. The Center provides parents with information on financial aid, recreational and social activities, and educational placement.

Part 4. THE TOTAL PICTURE (31 min, col)

This program is designed to provide the professional with special observational skills for dealing with the family in a home setting.

Part 5. PARENTS ARE PEOPLE FIRST (31 min, col)

Stresses the importance of family support for, and acceptance of a handicapped child.

Part 6. GENETIC COUNSELING: RURAL DELIVERY SYSTEM (27 min, b&w)

Discusses the problems of providing genetic counseling in rural areas.

Part 7. DIANA: ONE FAMILY'S EXPERIENCE (19 min, b&w)

The history of a multiply-handicapped child is presented by her parents. Problems in finding community services for Diana are discussed.

A FAMILY COPES WITH MALIGNANT UNCERTAINTY (1979, 3/4" videocassette, 42 min, col)
    Production: St. Louis Medical Center; Alice Dean Kitchen
    Distribution: St. Louis Medical Center, Audiovisual Department, $95
      for purchase; $25 for preview

Examines the effects of a life-threatening illness on a patient, and on family and friends in terms of their various perspectives, interpretations and roles. A couple, Ron and Cathy, discuss the behavioral disruption caused by a malignant brain tumor and stress the need for adjustment and acceptance of impending death.

THE FATHER (1970, 16mm film, 28 min, b&w)
    Production: Wabash Films and AFI
    Distribution: Michigan Media; $13.40 for rental

Portrays Ned Kelly, an aged New York cab driver who tries to discuss his son's recent death to his passengers. Burgess Meredith stars as this isolated and lonely man, searching for someone to share his grief. The program is an adaptation of the Chekov short story, "Grief."

THE FINAL, PROUD DAYS OF ELSIE WURSTER
    (see series: "To Age Is Human" - Part 1)

FINANCES/INSURANCE
    (see series: "Coping With Serious Illness" - Part 5)

FOUR WOMEN: BREAST CANCER (1979, 16mm film, 3/4" videocassette, 55 min, col)
    Production: Canadian Broadcasting Corporation
    Distribution: Filmakers Library; $650 for 16mm purchase; $500 for 3/4"
      purchase; $75 for 16mm rental

Four women who have undergone mastectomies discuss their fears before surgery, and their adjustment afterward.

FRITZI: LIVING AND DYING WITH DIGNITY   (1977, 3/4" videocassette, 50 min, col)
Production: Health and Education Multimedia, Inc.
Distribution: Audio Visual Medical Marketing, Inc.; $295 for purchase; $50 for rental

A patient is interviewed who is suffering from terminal breast cancer. The interview ranges from discussing dissatisfaction with health care providers and their difficulty in dealing with death, to the more theoretical yet practical implications of a Living Will. The husband of the patient joins the discussion in the last 15 minutes to provide his perspective on his wife's impending death.

FROM BOTH ENDS OF THE STETHOSCOPE   (1979, 3/4" or 1/2" videocassette, 38 min, col)
Production: Scripps Memorial Hospital Cancer Center; John S. Trumbold
Distribution: John S. Trumbold, Scripps Memorial Cancer Center Films

This program focuses on Dr. David Peters' struggle to live with cancer, not just die from it. The doctor-patient relationship is discussed, as are ways in which dealing with cancer can be improved. The program informs doctors of areas in which greater communication is needed. Dr. Peters noted that patients responded better to him once they learned of his vulnerability to illness. This interview was taped a few weeks before Peters, age thirty-eight died.

THE GENE ENGINEERS   (1977, 16mm film, 3/4" or 1/2" videocassette, 57 min, col)
Production: WGBH
Distribution: Time-Life Video; $700 for 16mm purchase; $200 for 3/4" purchase; $150 for 1/2" purchase; $60 for rental

This Nova program examines the potential scientific, ethical, and legal problems raised by developments in genetic manipulation. The program discusses possible benefits of new genetic combinations, but also questions their dangers.

THE GENETIC CHANCE   (1976, 3/4" videocassette, 57 min, col)
Production: BBC/WGBH
Distribution: King Features Entertainment, Inc.; $325 for purchase; $75 for rental

Examines many issues in the area of genetics and hereditary diseases. These issues include the following: hemophilia, sex determination, eugenic abortion, amniocentesis, civil rights, karotyping, quality of life, prognosis, and genetic counseling.

GENETIC COUNSELING: A PRACTICAL DEMONSTRATION OF A COUNSELING SESSION FOR
    PARENTS OF A DOWN'S SYNDROME CHILD (1978, 3/4" videocassette, 27 min,
    col)
    Production: University of Texas, Health Sciences Center at Dallas
    Distribution: Mrs. Esther Ruiz; $100 for purchase; $30 for rental

    Discusses genetic counseling methods.

GENETIC DEFECTS: THE BROKEN CODE (1976, 16mm film, 3/4", 1/2", or 1/4"
    videocassette, 57 min, col)
    Production: WNET, for PBS
    Distribution: Indiana University, Audio-Visual Center; $770 for 16mm,
    3/4", 1/2", or 1/4" purchase; $27.75 for 16mm rental

    Defines terminology in genetic studies, and explains mechanisms for pass-
    ing genetic diseases from generation to generation. The most common
    genetic defects in the U.S. population are then examined, such as: cys-
    tic fibrosis, Huntington's chorea, hemophilia, combined immune deficiency,
    and sickle cell disorder. This program also describes amniocentesis.

GENETIC ENGINEERING: LIFE IN OUR HANDS (1978, audiocassette, 59 min)
    Production: National Public Radio
    Distribution: National Public Radio; $7 for purchase

    Gerald Piel, publisher of Scientific American, lectures on genetic en-
    gineering. Using examples, he explores the question of whether scien-
    tists can maintain controls on genetic experiments.

GENETIC RESEARCH: ANOTHER GENIE IN A BOTTLE (1978, 2 filmstrips, 2 audio-
    cassettes or LP records, col, guide)
    Production: Audio Visual Narrative Arts, Inc.
    Distribution: Audio Visual Narrative Arts, Inc.; $69.50 for purchase

    The first filmstrip in this program outlines the basic chemistry behind
    the Watson-Crick model of DNA structure. The x-ray diffraction data
    which made inference of the double helical structure possible is also
    discussed. The second filmstrip analyzes social implications of genetic
    research, both in the future and at present.

GENETIC SCREENING (1979, audiocassette, 59 min)
    Production: National Public Radio
    Distribution: National Public Radio; $7 for purchase

    Participants discuss the capabilities, techniques, and aims of genetics
    as practiced today. They explain the various tests and social programs
    (e.g., screening programs for Tay Sachs and sickle-cell disorder) that

have become available as a result of these advances in genetic research. Panelists debate the moral dilemmas faced by religious communities, the government, and the lay person because of genetic screening.

GENETIC SCREENING: THE ULTIMATE IN PREVENTIVE MEDICINE?
(see series: "Hard Choices" - Part 2)

THE GERIATRIC PATIENT (1977, 3/4" videocassette, 15 min, col)
Production: Hugh J. Lurie
Distribution: The University of Washington Press; $175 for purchase

Eleven vignettes dealing with situations particular to geriatric patients are presented. The issues dealt with include: depression, loneliness, the feeling of being a burden, paranoia, senility, and conflicts about sexuality. The program is designed to stimulate discussion in the areas of interviewing techniques, intervention strategies, and diagnostic issues.

GRIEF THERAPY (1976, 16mm film, 3/4" videocassette, 19 min, col)
Production: CBS News
Distribution: Carousel (CBS) Films, Inc.; $375 for 16mm or 3/4" purchase; apply for rental information

A special treatment for intensely grief-stricken people is examined. Dr. Donald Ramsey of the University of Amsterdam is shown working with a mother who is still grieving two and a half years after her daughter's death. His ability to encourage her to accept her daughter's death is seen as successful.

THE GRIEVING PROCESS
(see series: "Terminal Illness" - Parts 5 & 6)

GROUP HOME LIVING: A MOVEMENT TOWARD INDEPENDENCE?
(see series: "Family and Its Relationship to the Develpmentally Disabled: Legal, Ethical, and Moral Issues" - Part 1)

GROWING OLD IN AMERICA (1980, 3/4" videocassette, 29 min, col)
Production: University of Michigan Media Resources Center
Distribution: Michigan Media; $25 for rental

Dorothy Coons, gerontologist, and Karen Mason, sociologist, interview May Sarton, author of the novel, As We Are Now. They discuss Sarton's experiences in nursing homes while researching for her book. The quality of life in such settings is described, and the importance of warmth and caring in these homes is emphasized.

HARD CHOICES (1980, series in 6 parts, 3/4" or 1/2" videocassette, each
    program 60 min, col, guide)
    Production: KCTS/Seattle
    Distribution: PBS Video; $1200 for 3/4" or 1/2" series purchase;
    $200 for 3/4" or 1/2" single program purchase; $70 for 3/4" single
    program rental

Part 1. BOY OR GIRL: SHOULD THE CHOICE BE OURS?

    Outlines prenatal testing procedures for determining the sex of a
    fetus. By using this knowledge, it may be possible to choose a baby's
    sex through selective abortion. Ethical questions raised by this pos-
    sibility are discussed.

Part 2. GENETIC SCREENING: THE ULTIMATE IN PREVENTIVE MEDICINE?

    Examines ethical questions raised by the practice of genetic screen-
    ing, such as who should decide what is considered a "normal" child.

Part 3. HUMAN EXPERIMENTS: THE PRICE OF KNOWLEDGE

    Analyzes the problem of protecting the rights and welfare of human
    subjects in medical research. Although the program acknowledges the
    need for experimentation in the search for medical knowledge, it
    weighs the costs and benefits of these experiments, to both society
    and the subjects involved.

Part 4. BEHAVIOR CONTROL

    This program questions the use of behavior control and its ethical
    ramifications, such as possible limits to autonomy and the right to
    self-determination.

Part 5. DEATH AND DYING

    Examines ways in which modern life-prolonging technology has compli-
    cated issues in death and dying. For example, when does a physician's
    responsibility to preserve life end, and when is a patient considered
    dead?

Part 6. DOCTOR, I WANT...

    Problems of health care allocation of scarce resources are examined.
    The program also includes discussion of the pros and cons of a na-
    tional health insurance program.

HAROLD
    (see series: "People You'd Like to Know" - Part 5)

HEALING (1977, 16mm film, 3/4" videocassette, 56 min, col)
   Production: National Film Board of Canada
   Distribution: Filmakers Library; $650 for 16mm purchase; $500 for
     3/4" purchase; $75 for 16mm rental

This documentary explores the phenomenon of faith healing in a modern-
day society. The program presents a demonstration of a celebrated
faith healer, Kathryn Kuhlman, as she exhibits her powers before a standing-
room only crowd in Canada. The reasons for faith healing's popularity,
its effectiveness and risks, are discussed.

HELP US HELP OURSELVES (early 1970s, 3/4" or 1/2" videocassette, 25 min,
   col)
   Production: Medix
   Distribution: The Trainex Health Care Library; $295 for 3/4" or 1/2"
     purchase; $55 for 3/4" rental

Individuals who are successfully adapting to physical disabilities are
featured in this program. Participants in the program include: Jill
Kinmont, a former national skiing champion, Gary Green, a Vietnam vet-
eran and amputee jet pilot, and a group of one-legged snow skiers.

HOSPICE (1976, 16mm film, 38 min, col)
   Production: Behr Cinemetography
   Distribution: Michigan Media; $33.20 for rental

Profiles the services and philosophy of St. Christopher's Hospice in
England.

HOSPICE ENCOUNTERS AND MENTAL HEALTH TRAINING FILM (1981, 3/4", 1/2",
   or 1/4" videocassette, 17 min, col)
   Production: Berkley Hospice Training Project
   Distribution: Berkley Hospice Training Project; $150 for purchase;
     apply for rental information

Designed for use by discussion groups in the training of hospice professionals, this program teaches counseling techniques using a hospice
setting.

HOSPITAL (1970, 16mm film, 84 min, b&w)
   Production: Frederick Wiseman
   Distribution: Zipporah Films; $1200 for 5-year lease; $150 for rental

Portrays a metropolitan hospital's daily routine and tragedies. There
is no narrative or commentary; the problems of the people and the hospital are self-evident.

HOW COULD I NOT BE AMONG YOU? (1972, 16mm film, 28 min, col)
    Production: Thomas Reichman
    Distribution: Benchmark Films, Inc.; $525 for purchase; $55 for
      rental

    This film portrays a thirty-two-year-old poet, Ted Rosenthal, who is dying
    of leukemia. His last months of life are shown, and his anticipation of
    death is documented in this period.

HOW OLD ARE YOU NOW? (1976, audiocassette, 59 min)
    Production: National Public Radio
    Distribution: National Public Radio; $7 for purchase

    Seven people discuss their belief systems, their work, and how they
    deal with their own mortality. Persons described as a minister, a poet,
    a biologist, an American Indian, and a humanist contribute to this discussion
    on death.

HUMAN EXPERIMENTS: THE PRICE OF KNOWLEDGE?
    (see series: "Hard Choices" - Part 5)

HUMANISM IN HEALTH CARE (1979, 3/4" videocassette, 34 min, col)
    Production: Emory University School of Medicine
    Distribution: Emory Medical Television Network; $120 for purchase;
      $35 for rental

    Examines humanistic care in the hospital setting. The program closes
    with a slide-audiocassette segment based on the poem, "What Do You See?,"
    written by a geriatric patient.

I AM NOT WHAT YOU SEE (1978, 16mm film, 3/4" videocassette, 28 min, col)
    Production: Canadian Broadcasting Corporation
    Distribution: Filmakers Library; $425 for 16mm purchase; $375 for
      3/4" purchase; $45 for 16mm rental

    A severely crippled cerebral palsy victim, Sondra Diamond, is featured
    in this program. Despite her physical handicap - she is confined to a
    wheelchair and is unable to perform routine tasks such as dressing or
    bathing - she is a practicing psychologist, and works for the rights
    of the handicapped. Ms. Diamond's determination is strong, and she
    believes every human being has the right to live, disabled or not.

I'M STILL THE SAME PERSON (1980, 3/4" videocassette, 29 min, col)
    Production: University of Michigan Media Resources Center
    Distribution: Michigan Media; $25 for rental

    This program features two high-school students, Jenny Miller and Bob

Fascetti, who have contracted and undergone treatment for cancer. They discuss their feelings about cancer, the reactions of their families and friends, and their plans for the future.

IN RE ACKROYD (1978, 3/4" videocassette, 150 min, col)
Production: Concern for Dying
Distribution: Concern for Dying; $200 for purchase; $40 for rental

A mock trial of a case involving the withdrawal of life support from a comatose, irreversibly brain-damaged man. The trial is adlibbed by real health care professionals, and the verdict is left to the viewer. The clinical, legal, and ethical dilemmas raised in this case are realistic.

IN VITRO FERTILIZATION (1979, audiocassette, 59 min)
Production: National Public Radio
Distribution: National Public Radio; $7 for purchase

Panelists discuss the procedure of in vitro fertilization and examine causes of infertility. Other topics discussed in this program include: the need for laws governing ownership of stored sperm and eggs, moral dilemmas, and medical dangers.

INTERVIEWS WITH THE PATIENT
(see series: "Terminal Illness" - Part 1)

THE ISSUE OF CONFIDENTIALITY AND MEDICAL RECORDS (1976, audiocassette, 18 min)
Production: Communications in Learning
Distribution: Communications in Learning; $15.95 for purchase

Ethical issues of confidentiality and medical records are discussed in this program. Topics include: privileged communication, physician-patient relationship, information retrieval systems, medical records, and truth-telling.

JAMES IS OUR BROTHER (1979, 16mm film, 3/4" or 1/2" videocassette, 22 min, col)
Production: BBC
Distribution: Time-Life Video; $350 for 16mm purchase; $200 for 3/4" purchase; $150 for 1/2" purchase; $30 for rental

A profile of James, a sixteen-year-old boy who is a mongoloid. He will be graduated from his remedial school, and hopes to lead as normal a life as possible. He discusses life as a mentally retarded person, and his feelings about the way others view him.

JOAN ROBINSON: ONE WOMAN'S STORY (1980, 3/4" or 1/2" videocassette, 165 min, col)
   Production: Red Cloud Productions
   Distribution: Time-Life Video; $500 for 3/4" purchase; $400 for 1/2" purchase; $50 for rental

This is a record of Joan Robinson's twenty-two-month battle with cancer, before she finally died in 1975. All stages of Mrs. Robinson's illness and her responses to it are documented in this program, including questioning, fear, resolution, rage and transcendence. (The series, "Coping with Serious Illness," was adapted from this documentary.)

JOCELYN (1980, 16mm film, 3/4" videocassette, 28 min, col)
   Production: Canadian Broadcasting Corporation
   Distribution: Filmakers Library; $425 for 16mm purchase; $375 for 3/4" purchase; $45 for 16mm rental

A program about a seventeen-year-old girl facing imminent death. The program focuses on Jocelyn's life, rather than on the suffering of her dying. The emotional strength of Jocelyn, her family, and her friends, is emphasized.

JOEY (1977, 16mm film, 3/4" or 1/2" videocassette, 70 min, col)
   Production: BBC
   Distribution: Time-Life Video; $800 for 16mm purchase; $200 for 3/4" purchase; $150 for 1/2" purchase; $75 for rental

This program is about a man, Joey Desmond, who was born in 1920 with severe brain damage and grew up spastic. Institutionalized in 1928, he was unable to make himself understood. In 1941 he met a man, Ernie, who could understand him. Although Ernie was classified as an imbecile, thirty years later Joey dictated his memories to Ernie, who then dictated them to another man who could barely write. Two years later, Tongue Tied was published. Joey and Ernie play themselves in this true story.

JOHN
   (see series: "People You'd Like to Know" - Part 6)

KAI
   (see series: "People You'd Like to Know" - Part 7)

THE LAST DAYS OF LIVING (1980, 16mm film, 3/4" videocassette, 58 min, col)
   Production: National Film Board of Canada
   Distribution: National Film Board of Canada; $630 for 16mm purchase; $420 for 3/4" purchase; $60 for 16mm or 3/4" rental

Illustrates the efforts of the palliative care service at the Royal Victoria Hospital in Montreal to prepare a dying individual for death in a caring environment. A humanistic approach to meeting the needs of terminally ill patients and their families, modeled on the hospice concept, is demonstrated. Institutional death, societal attitudes toward death, pain control, appropriate therapy, the conspiracy of silence, and psychological issues are discussed. Living each day fully is advocated and contrasted to the inevitability of death. Interdisciplinary cooperation between various health care team members is reviewed and the current balance between comfort and treatment is emphasized.

LAST RITES (1979, 16mm film, 30 min, col)
    Production: Joan Vail Thorne, Anne Macksoud
    Distribution: Filmakers Library; $425 for purchase; $45 for rental

    Set in the early 1930s, this film examines a young boy's reaction to his mother's death. His transition from denial to acceptance and understanding of his mother's death is presented.

THE LIFE THAT'S LEFT (1978, 16mm film, 3/4" or 1/2" videocassette, 29 min, col)
    Production: Great Plains National Instructional Television Library
    Distribution: Great Plains National Instructional Television Library; $450 for 16mm purchase; $180 for 3/4" or 1/2" purchase; $40 for 16mm rental; $30 for 3/4" or 1/2" rental

    A collection of interviews with various individuals who have suffered the loss of a loved one: an elderly widower, a young mother bereaved of her husband, a teenager who has lost his brother, the parents of sons who died, and a young woman whose second child was stillborn.

LIKE OTHER PEOPLE (1973, 16mm film, 3/4", 1/2", or 1/4" videocassette, 37 min, col)
    Production: Kastrel, for Mental Health Film Council, England
    Distribution: Perennial Education, Inc.; $442 for 16mm purchase; $398 for 3/4", 1/2", or 1/4" purchase; $52 for 16mm rental

    Presents two cerebral palsy patients, Margaret and Willie, who are living in a home for the palsied in England. They discuss the needs of the handicapped in society, and their desire to marry and care for each other.

LITTLE CITY (1980, 16mm film, 3/4" videocassette, 30 min, col)
    Production: Alan Dachman
    Distribution: Filmakers Library; $425 for 16mm purchase; $375 for 3/4" purchase; $45 for 16mm rental

This program features the residents of Little City, a home, school and training center for mentally retarded children and adults. The emphasis of Little City is to prepare residents for life in the outside world by introducing them to social attitudes and skills necessary for independence.

LIVING TIME - SARAH JESUP TALKS ON DYING (1979, 16mm film, 15 min, col)
    Production: Concern for Dying
    Distribution: Concern for Dying; $150 for purchase; $25 for rental

A film about Sarah Jesup, who at forty-one years of age has three months to live. She discusses (only three weeks before her death) central issues of the dying patient's experience. She discusses her approach to explaining death to her children and friends. She also talks about the doctor-patient relationship, and her thoughts about the Living Will.

THE LONG VALLEY: A STUDY OF BEREAVEMENT (1978, 16mm film, 3/4" or 1/2"
    videocassette, 59 min, col)
    Production: BBC and OECA
    Distribution: Time-Life Video; $700 for 16mm purchase; $200 for 3/4"
      purchase; $150 for 1/2" purchase; $65 for rental

Presents Mr. Colin M. Parkes, a social psychiatrist, as he discusses the process of grief with a group of doctors, clergy, social workers, and bereaved people. Dr. Parkes discusses four stages of grief; shock and numbness, searching for the dead person, depression, and acceptance of death. The program emphasizes that our reactions to death should not be suppressed, because they are necessary and natural responses.

THE LOST PHOEBE (1978, 16mm film, 3/4" or 1/2" videocassette, 30 min, col)
    Production: American Film Institute
    Distribution: Coronet/Perspective Films; $519 for 16mm purchase; $311
      for 3/4" or 1/2" purchase

A remake of Theodore Dreiser's short story, "The Lost Phoebe," a tale of grief. Seventy year old Henry Reifsnyder is seen mourning the death of his wife of forty years, Phoebe. His grief becomes an obsession, before finally joining her in death himself in this story of unreconciled grief.

THE MALADY OF HEALTH CARE (1980, 16mm film, 3/4" or 1/2" videocassette,
    57 min, col)
    Production: WGBH
    Distribution: Time-Life Video; $750 for 16mm purchase; $200 for 3/4"
      purchase; $150 for 1/2" purchase; $75 for rental

A comparative study of British and United States health care delivery. The British National Health Service is contrasted with the United States' private health care system. This program raises problems of allocating scarce resources, such as whether limited funding should be used for creating more sophisticated technology, or for public health programs.

MARK
   (see series: "People You'd Like to Know" - Part 8)

MARY
   (see series: "People You'd Like to Know" - Part 9)

MEDICAL ETHICS (1977, 3/4" videocassette, 30 min, col)
   Production: WNED-TV, Buffalo, New York
   Distribution: American Humanist Association; $175 for purchase; $39
     for rental

   Louis Lasagna, Robert M. Veatch, and Paul Kurtz are featured in this
   survey of many issues of medical ethics. The issues include: physician-
   patient relationship, paternalism in health care, patient participation
   in decision-making, patient care, patient self-determination, informed
   consent, truth-telling, risks and benefits, and values.

MEDICAL-LEGAL ASPECTS OF AMNIOCENTESIS FOR PRENATAL DIAGNOSIS (1978, 16mm
   film, 3/4" videocassette, 14 min, col)
   Production: National Library of Medicine, National Audiovisual Center,
     in association with the Centers for Disease Control, Bureau of Epidemi-
     ology, Chronic Diseases Division, Birth Defects Branch
   Distribution: National Medical Audiovisual Center, c/o Modern Talking
     Pictures Service, Inc.; $10 for rental

   Medical, legal and ethical issues involved in amniocentesis and prenatal
   diagnosis are examined.

MISS LARSEN: REBEL AT 90 (1976, 16mm film, 17 min, col)
   Production: Herbert Danska
   Distribution: Michigan Media; $13.50 for rental

   This film, excerpted from "Nobody Ever Died of Old Age," presents the
   struggle of a ninety-year-old woman to preserve her dignity in nursing
   home and hospital situations. The film records ways in which the elderly
   can be degraded and treated like children.

MORE THAN A PLACE TO DIE
   (see series: "To Age Is Human" - Part 3)

THE MOURNING PROCESS: MRS. KELLY (1979, 3/4" videocassette, 51 min, col)
   Production: St. Louis Medical Center, Audiovisual Department, Alice
     Dean Kitchen
   Distribution: St. Louis Medical Center, Audiovisual Department; $95
     for purchase; $25 for rental

Features an interview with a woman, Mrs. Kelly, who is grieving the loss
of her husband. Three stages of grief: shock and disbelief, painful
emergence, and resolution, are characterized. (This program was produced
in conjunction with "Slow Death: Mr. and Mrs. Kelly.")

THE NATURE OF ETHICAL PROBLEMS (1980, slide and audiocassette, 24 min, col,
    guide)
    Production: Concept Media; Janet Freebairn, Karen Gwinup
    Distribution: Concept Media; $98 for purchase

    Part of a series on ethics in nursing. The program presents two major
    ethical theories, the teleological and deontological. A six-step model
    for analyzing ethical problems is presented.

A NEED TO KNOW: A FAMILY FACES DEATH (1976, 3/4" or 1/2" videocassette,
    60 min, col or b&w)
    Production: Lois Jaffe
    Distribution: Boston Family Institute; $275 for 3/4" or 1/2" purchase;
        $99 for 3/4" or 1/2" rental

    Presented in the format of a group session, this program illustrates from
    different angles the effect of an adolescent boy's leukemia on the family
    and on the marriage. A number of seldom spoken but critical factors are
    discussed candidly by the family, such as: feelings of guilt on the part
    of the parents, anger toward the physician who gives the final diagnosis,
    resentment on the part of the siblings, and the desire of the ill son to
    be treated as a normal person as much as possible.

NEVER TOO LATE
    (see series: "To Age Is Human" - Part 4)

THE NEW GENETICS: RIGHTS AND RESPONSIBILITIES
    (see series: "Science and Society" - Part 2)

NURSING OBLIGATIONS (1980, slide and audiocassette, 17 min, col)
    Production: Concept Media; Janet Freebairn, Karen Gwinup
    Distribution: Concept Media; $98 for purchase

    Discusses ethical issues involved in secret-keeping, confidentiality, and
    professionalism. The responsibilities of nurses when they are not working
    as nurses are also discussed.

OLD MYTHS, NEW REALITIES
    (see series: "To Age Is Human" - Part 5)

ONE OF OUR OWN (1980, 16mm film, 55 min, col)
  Production: Canadian Broadcasting Corporation
  Distribution: Filmakers Library; $700 for purchase; $75 for rental

  David McFarlane, the boy presented in the film, "David," plays a retarded
  boy approaching maturity. His family is concerned about the wisdom of
  keeping him at home any longer as they move to a new community. He manages
  to adjust to the new community, however, and he realizes that he can learn
  skills that will enable him to become independent.

ONE, TWO, THREE, ZERO: INFERTILITY (1980, 16mm film, 3/4" videocassette,
  28 min, col)
  Production: Canadian Broadcasting Corporation
  Distribution: Filmakers Library; $425 for 16mm purchase; $375 for 3/4"
    purchase; $45 for 16mm rental

  Presents six couples who have sought help from the fertility clinic of
  the Toronto General Hospital. Advances in modern medicine that have
  helped such couples are discussed. The emotional strain infertility
  places on a couple is examined, as are the legal and ethical ramifica-
  tions of certain treatments, such as surrogate parentage and test-tube
  pregnancies.

THE OTHER GENERATION GAP (1978, audiocassette, 59 min)
  Production: National Public Radio
  Distribution: National Public Radio; $7 for purchase

  Dr. Steven Cohen, author of The Other Generation Gap: The Middle-Aged
  and Their Aging Parents, discusses responsibility for one's parents,
  and emphasizes distinguishing between a parent's needs and wants. Maggie
  Kuhn, founder of the Grey Panthers, talks about the media's portrayal of
  older people, the demographic changes of society, the use of drugs to
  ease the pain of dying, and the problems of older people in nursing homes.

PAIGE
  (see series: "People You'd Like to Know" - Part 10)

PAIN
  (see series: "Coping with Serious Illness" - Part 1)

PAIN MANAGEMENT
  (see series: "Terminal Illness" - Part 3)

PARENT POWER: A LOOK AT THE PARENT INFORMATION CENTER OF CINCINNATI
  (see series: "The Family and Its Relationship to the Developmentally
  Disabled: Legal, Ethical, and Moral Issues" - Part 3)

PARENTS AND CHILDREN (1977, 16mm film, 3/4" videocassette, 30 min, col,
   guide)
   Production: American Journal of Nursing Co.
   Distribution: American Journal of Nursing Co. (New York) for purchase;
      American Journal of Nursing Co., Videotape Library (Chicago) for
      rental; $395 for 16mm purchase; $265 for 3/4" purchase; $35 for
      16mm rental; $30 for 3/4" rental

   Examines the status of legal minors with regard to: informed consent,
   consent of parents with minor children, the differences between the
   emergency situation and the usual treatment situation, state laws covering abortion for minors, role of the parents in abortion for minors, and
   the legal and ethical role of the nurse in child abuse and wife beating.

PARENTS ARE PEOPLE FIRST
   (see series: "The Family and Its Relationship to the Developmentally
      Disabled: Legal, Ethical, and Moral Issues" - Part 5)

PASSING QUIETLY THROUGH (1970, 16mm film, 26 min, b&w)
   Production: Dinitia Smith McCarthy
   Distribution: Grove Press; $325 for purchase; $30 for rental

   Examines the relationship between a geriatric patient and a nurse,
   focusing on the emotional aspects of their interaction.

PATIENT AUTONOMY (1980, slide and audiocassette, 21 min, col, guide)
   Production: Concept Media; Janet Freebairn, Karen Gwinup
   Distribution: Concept Media; $98 for purchase

   Discusses ways in which health care personnel neglect patient autonomy.
   Issues of paternalism, coercion vs. informed consent, and truth-telling
   are examined.

A PATIENT'S BILL OF RIGHTS (1980, slide and audiocassette, 25 min, col,
   guide)
   Production: Concept Media; Janet Freebairn, Karen Gwinup
   Distribution: Concept Media; $98 for purchase

   Outlines the twelve provisions of the American Hospital Association's
   statement on patient's rights. Interpretation of these provisions is
   provided by an authority on patient's rights. Problems of implementing
   these rights are discussed, as well as the role of the nurse as patient
   advocate in insuring that these rights are not violated.

PEEGE (1974, 16mm film, 3/4", 1/2", or 1/4" videocassette, 28 min, col)
   Production: David Knapp
   Distribution: Phoenix Films, Inc.; $465 for 16mm purchase; $315 for
      3/4", 1/2", or 1/4" purchase; $40 for 16mm purchase.

This film depicts a family's response to a Christmas Eve visit to grandma, or Peege. She is in a custodial care home, blind, unable to sit upright, control her bowels, feed herself, or remember events and people most of the time. Each family member reveals his or her character in this encounter. The only member of the family able to respond to Peege as a human being is the eldest son. When the rest of the family has departed after their awkward visit, the elder son stays behind to talk to Peege. As he leaves, her face lights up in recognition of a memory he has sparked in his attempts to communicate with her as a person. The film highlights changes in American family structure and society which have allowed distancing and isolation of elderly relatives.

THE PEOPLE YOU NEVER SEE (1978, 16mm film, 3/4" videocassette, 28 min, col)
Production: Canadian Broadcasting Corporation
Distribution: Filmakers Library; $425 for 16mm purchase; $375 for 3/4"
    purchase; $45 for 16mm rental

Presents several young people with cerebral palsy who have managed to live in mainstream society. Problems of access for the physically handicapped are highlighted by attempts of these young people to live independent lives.

PEOPLE YOU'D LIKE TO KNOW (1978, series in 10 parts, 16mm film, 3/4", 1/2",
or 1/4" videocassette, each program 10 min, col)
Production: WGBH/Encyclopedia Brittanica Educational Corporation
Distribution: Encyclopedia Brittanica Educational Corporation; $1680
    for 16mm, 3/4", 1/2", or 1/4" series purchase; $205 for 16mm, 3/4",
    1/2", or 1/4" single program purchase; $14 for 16mm, 3/4", 1/2", or
    1/4" single program rental

Features ten children, ages 11-14 years old, with various disabilities. Methods for coping with handicaps are stressed in this series.

Part 1. C.J.

This program features C.J.,an emotionally disturbed youth.

Part 2. DEE

Dee is a twelve year old girl who was born with Larson's syndrome. She spends half of each day in a school for the handicapped, and the other half in a school with non-handicapped children. Feelings about mainstreaming are presented in this program.

Part 3. DIANA

A program about Diana, who has had one leg amputated because of bone cancer.

Part 4. ELIZABETH

Elizabeth suffers from low vision, yet is mainstreamed for all of her junior high school classes.

Part 5. HAROLD

Harold is a fourteen year old boy who is blind, yet is mainstreamed for all of his classes.

Part 6. JOHN

This program features a fourteen year old boy, John, who has cystic fibrosis.

Part 7. KAI

Kai is a junior high school student who came to the United States four years ago, and who was born with a cleft lip and palate.

Part 8. MARK

Mark, a fourteen year old boy with a learning disability, explains his difficulties.

Part 9. MARY

Mary is an eleven year old girl with impaired hearing and speech. She attends public school, however, and participates in extracurricular activities.

Part 10. PAIGE

Paige was born with Down's Syndrome. The eleven year old spends part of her day in a resource room, and part in a regular fourth grade class.

PERSON TO PERSON: THE AACP/ELI LILLY PHARMACY SKILLS PROJECT, VOLUME ONE:
   EMPATHY (1981, 3/4" videocassette, 30 min, col, guide)
   Production: Northeastern University College of Pharmacy and Allied Health
      Professions and Office of Learning Resources; David Barnard, Judith Barr,
      Gerald Schumacher
   Distribution: Available on loan from Continuing Education Departments of
      local colleges of pharmacy

Illustrates empathetic behavior in clinical pharmacy situations, and dis-cusses the major components of empathetic listening and response. Accurate listening and perception, recognition of personal biases and distortions, and an attitude of genuinely prizing the human qualities of patients and clients are described and illustrated with dramatizations from pharmacy practice.

PERSPECTIVES ON DEATH (1976, 2 filmstrips and audiocassettes)
    Production: Sunburst Communications
    Distribution: Sunburst Communications; $89 for series purchase

    Part 1. TOWARD AN ACCEPTANCE

        Examines different attitudes toward death, and emphasizes the need to
        view death as a part of life.

    Part 2. THE RIGHT TO DIE

        Explores social problems caused by advances in medical technology.
        Ethical issues surrounding euthanasia - both active and passive -
        are discussed.

PINS AND NEEDLES (1980, 16mm film, 3/4" videocassette, 37 min, col)
    Production: Genni Batterham, Kim Batterham
    Distribution: Filmakers Library; $450 for 16mm purchase; $400 for
        3/4" purchase; $45 for 16mm rental

    This film portrays Genni Batterham who has multiple sclerosis. She is
    a young, married, successful woman, who has maintained her sense of
    purpose and dignity despite her disability. Her fears of losing her
    husband as a result of her illness are voiced. She also criticizes
    society's neglect of the handicapped. Among the issues discussed in the
    film are: sexuality, self-esteem, dependency, denial of reality by family,
    the appropriateness of occupational workshops, and the problems of access.

A PLAGUE ON OUR CHILDREN (1980, 2 programs, 16mm film, 3/4" or 1/2" video-
    cassette, each program 57 min, col)
    Production: WGBH
    Distribution: Time-Life Video; $700 for 16mm single program purchase;
        $200 for 3/4" single program purchase; $150 for 1/2" single program
        purchase; $65 for single program rental

    Part 1. DIOXINS

        Discusses health hazards of dioxin defoliants such as Sylvex sprayed
        on Oregon forests and Agent Orange dropped on Vietnam. The program
        argues that Dioxins are responsible for miscarriages, cancers, and
        disease, because Dioxin molecules fit into the basic DNA structure,
        altering it and causing mutations.

    Part 2. PCBs

        The problem of cleaning up toxic chemical waste is examined in this
        program. Love Canal, New York, is shown as an example of dangerous
        and irresponsible handling of toxic wastes. After leaks were dis-
        covered in drums of toxic waste dumped by the Hooker Chemical and

Plastic Company, several hundred residents of Love Canal were evacuated permanently from their homes. The program notes that adequate methods have not been found to break down the non-biodegradable structure of PCBs.

PLEASE LET ME DIE (1974, 3/4" videocassette, 30 min, col)
    Production: University of Texas Medical Branch at Galveston; Dr. Robert
    B. White
    Distribution: Dr. Robert B. White; $150 for purchase; $50 for rental

Features a young man who was burned over 70% of his body, leaving him blind and severely maimed. The filming for this program takes place ten months after his accident. At issue is the treatment he continues to receive and his desire to end treatment and die. Graphic footage of his burns is included, as well as a discussion between the patient and a psychiatrist. (Available to limited audiences; inquire for information about distribution requirements).

PRE-NATAL DIAGNOSIS (1981, 16mm film, 3/4" videocassette, 45 min, col)
    Production: Canadian Broadcasting Corporation
    Distribution: Filmakers Library; $575 for 16mm purchase; $500 for
    3/4" purchase; $65 for 16mm rental

New methods for detecting birth defects are presented in this program, such as amniocentesis, fetoscopy, and ultrasound. Ethical questions raised by prenatal diagnosis are raised, questions for both doctors and parents. These include the problem of deciding whether to terminate a pregnancy because of defects and whether to test for sex or for physical characteristics such as cleft palate.

PSYCHOLOGIAL ASPECTS OF DEATH (1971, 16mm film, 3/4", 1/2", or 1/4" video-
    cassette, 39 min, b&w)
    Production: Indiana University School of Nursing
    Distribution: Indiana University, Audio-Visual Center; $300 for 16mm
    purchase; $200 for 3/4", 1/2", or 1/4" purchase; $11.25 for 16mm
    rental

Presents a dramatization in which a man and his wife are suddenly confronted with the psychological aspects of dying. Johnny Wilson, a leukemia patient, is admitted to the hospital for "routine tests" for a chest cold. He discusses with a nurse and his pregnant wife his desires to help support the family, rather than staying at home. Unexpectedly, Johnny suffers a cardiac arrest and dies. The nurse overcomes her personal grief in order to comfort Johnny's wife and mother-in-law.

PSYCHOLOGICAL REACTIONS OF THE DYING PERSON (1972, filmstrip and audio-
cassette, 30 min, col, guide)
Production: Concept Media; Karen Gwinup, Donna C. Aguilera
Distribution: Concept Media; $98 for purchase

Pictures of people are used to depict psychological reactions of the
dying person. The manner in which a person responds to a fatal illness
is explored. The individual's personal characteristics, interpersonal
relationships, particularly those with his or her family, and the nature
of the illness as it influences the patient's responses are examined. The
grief process and two different types of psychological responses - coping
mechanisms and emotional reactions - are explained. Implications for
nursing care of the dying patient are underscored in this discussion. The
dying person's final state of mind and the factors which influence his
ability to accept his death are described.

THE QUANTITY AND QUALITY OF LIFE (1979, audiocassette, 59 min)
Production: National Public Radio
Distribution: National Public Radio; $7 for purchase

Dr. Christian Barnard, South African heart specialist, and Representative
Richardson Preyer (D., N.C.), member of the House Health Subcommittee,
discuss modern health care. Dr. Barnard explains that the goal of medicine should be to improve the overall quality of a patient's life, not just
to prolong it. Representative Preyer emphasizes the importance of con-
trolling medical technology without hampering scientific research. Both
consider the issues of the "right to life," the financing of health care,
and curative vs. preventative medicine.

A QUESTION OF VALUES (1973, 16mm film, 3/4", 1/2", or 1/4" videocassette,
24 min, col)
Production: Edward Feil Productions
Distribution: Edward Feil Productions; $259 for 16mm, 3/4", 1/2", or
1/4" purchase; $25 for 16mm rental

This film was inspired by the Kennedy Foundation's production, "Who Should
Survive?," in which a Down's Syndrome child was allowed to die. "A
Question of Values" presents information about Down's Syndrome, and features three Down's children, one of whom had been treated for the same intestinal blockage that was left untreated in the Kennedy film. Legal and
philosophical issues of treating or withholding treatment for potentially
dependent persons are examined in this program. (These two films are sometimes shown together).

RECOMBINANT D.N.A. (1978, audiocassette, 59 min)
Production: National Public Radio
Distribution: National Public Radio; $7 for purchase

Professionals discuss the moral and legal problems posed by gene-splicing
(recombinant D.N.A.). They talk about the safety factors and the research
guidelines of the National Institutes of Health.

RELATIONSHIPS
    (see series: "Coping with Serious Illness" - Part 4)

RELIGION AND THE CLERGY
    (see series: "Terminal Illness" - Part 4)

REMOVING LIFE SUPPORT (1977, 3/4" videocassette, 25 min, col)
    Production: Creighton University School of Medicine
    Distribution: Learning Resources Center, Bio-Information Center,
      Creighton University; $11.50 for rental

    Discusses the ethical problems involved in the doctor's or family's
    decision to remove life support systems.

THE RIGHT TO DIE (1974, 16mm film, 56 min, col)
    Production: American Broadcasting Co.; Marlene Sanders
    Distribution: MacMillan Films, Inc.; $660 for purchase; $55 for rental

    Examines conflicts in dying, such as when technological prolongation of
    life should be withheld. The program includes interviews with dying
    patients, and discussion of the ways in which family, medical personnel,
    and clergy deal with death and dying. Patients are presented who express
    a desire to know of their condition in order to be prepared for death.

THE RIGHT TO LET DIE (1973, 16mm film, 28 min, col)
    Production: Joseph P. Kennedy, Jr. Foundation
    Distribution: Lowengard & Brotherhood; $190 for purchase; $25 for
      rental

    A panel discussion which examines central ethical questions of the right
    to let a patient die. The panel includes: David C. Abramson, M.D., Ph.D.,
    Director of Newborn Services, Georgetown; Sydney Cornelia Callahan, M.A.,
    L.L.D., author and columnist, Hastings-on-Hudson; Warren T. Reich, S.T.D.,
    Kennedy Center for Bioethics, Georgetown.

THE RIGHT TO LIVE: WHO DECIDES? (1972, 16mm film, 3/4", 1/2", or 1/4"
    videocassette, 15 min, b&w)
    Production: Hanley Thomson
    Distribution: Learning Corporation of America; $270 for 16mm purchase;
      $200 for 3/4", 1/2", or 1/4" videocassette; $30 for 16mm, 3/4", 1/2",
      or 1/4" rental

    An excerpt from Columbia Picture's "Abandon Ship," starring Tyrone Power
    as the commanding officer of a lifeboat rescuing passengers of a sinking
    ship. During a storm it becomes apparent that not all of the passengers
    can stay aboard if any are to survive. The question of who shall live
    and who shall perish in this situation is raised. It offers a discussion
    parallel for such decision-making in the hospital setting.

RIGHTS OF PATIENTS (mid-1970s, 16mm film, 3/4" videocassette, 60 min, col, guide)
Production: American Journal of Nursing Co.
Distribution: American Journal of Nursing Co. (New York) for purchase; American Journal of Nursing Co., Videotape Library (Chicago) for rental; $395 for 16mm purchase; $265 for 3/4" purchase; $35 for 16mm rental; $30 for 3/4" rental

A number of issues in patient's rights are examined, including: the right to information, informed consent, refusal of care, incapacitated patients who are minors, emergencies, treatment by students, experimentation, privacy, ownership of records, and protection from unprofessional conduct. Vignettes are used to depict many of these situations.

THE ROLE OF THE PHYSICIAN
(see series: "Terminal Illness" - Part 2)

THE SCIENCE AND ETHICS OF POPULATION CONTROL: AN OVERBURDENED EARTH?
(1975, slide and audiocassette, 32 min, col, guide)
Production: Science and Mankind, Inc.
Distribution: Science and Mankind, Inc.; $159.50 for purchase

Examines ethical problems raised by the following topics: population growth, food shortages, public policy, social control, population control, poverty, developing countries, survival, economics, involuntary sterilization, coercion, and medical technology.

SCIENCE AND SOCIETY (1974-'76, series in 3 parts, slide and audiocassette, col, guide)
Production: Science and Mankind, Inc.
Distribution: Science and Mankind, Inc.; $299.70 for series purchase; $169.50 for single program purchase

Part 1. THE ETHICS OF GENETIC CONTROL (1976, 37 min)

Examines the following topics: Eugenics, discrimination, gene pools, hereditary diseases, prenatal diagnosis, coercion, genetic screening, reproduction, human rights, social control, social problems, fertilization in vitro, sex determination, the embryo, amniocentesis, eugenic abortion, quality of life, and decision-making.

Part 2. THE NEW GENETICS: RIGHTS AND RESPONSIBILITIES (1974, 47 min)
Examines the following topics: genetic screening and counseling, decision-making, reproduction, civil rights, social control, cost benefit analysis, genetic intervention, hereditary disease, physician's responsibilities, recessive genes, heterozygotes, coercion, risk, central nervous system diseases, phenylketonuria, economics, amniocentesis, eugenic abortion, dominant genes.

Part 3. THE ETHICAL CHALLENGE: FOUR BIOMEDICAL CASE STUDIES (1975, 32 min)

Problems in biomedical practice are examined through four case studies. The studies examine: scarce medical resources, behavior control, genetic screening, and the question of when to terminate life-prolonging treatment and who should make that decision.

SCIENCE AND SOCIETY: RECONCILING TWO PERSPECTIVES (1975, 6 filmstrips and audiocassettes, 12-15 min each, col, guide)
Production: Jacoby/Storm Productions
Distribution: Sunburst Communications; $169 for series purchase; 30-day free loan

Examines the following topics: science, social values, medicine, social responsibility, medical technology, religion, genetics, humanities, jurisprudence, research, government financing, social control, human experimentation, human rights, genetic intervention, economics, population control, food shortages, bioethics, and government.

SCIENTIFIC MEDICINE: TECHNOLOGY AND THE CONCEPT OF HEALTH (1977, 3/4" videocassette, 46 min, col)
Production: Creighton University School of Medicine
Distribution: Learning Resources Center, Bio-Information Center, Creighton University; $11.50 for rental

Presents a discussion of medical technology, behavior and genetic control, and the concept of "health" in general.

SECRETS (1980, 16mm film, 8 min, col)
Production: Joan Vail Thorne, Bill Richards
Distribution: Filmakers Library; $200 for purchase; $30 for rental

This program serves to remind the viewer that stereotyping the elderly is impossible. An eighty-year-old businessman is shown during the course of a working day, and the "secrets" and mysteries in his life reveal an energetic and full life.

SEXUALITY
(see series: "Coping with Serious Illness" - Part 3)

SHOULD PASSIVE EUTHANASIA BE PERMITTED? (1977, audiocassette, 13 min)
Production: Tom McCall, Laurence V. Foye
Distribution: Greenhaven Press; $5.98 for purchase

Examines the following topics: passive euthanasia, the aged, wills, pain, life-support, extraordinary treatment, and physician's responsibilities.

SLOW DEATH: MR. AND MRS. KELLY (1979, 3/4" videocassette, 45 min, col)
 Production: St. Louis University Medical Center, Audiovisual Department; Alice Dean Kitchen
 Distribution: St. Louis University Medical Center, Audiovisual Department; $95 for purchase; $25 for rental

 Portrays the slow, debilitating illness of a sixty-five-year-old man.
 His spouse's response to long-term care, the opinion of the visiting
 nurse, and the commentary of a psychiatrist are included. (This program
 was produced in conjunction with "The Mourning Process: Mrs. Kelly.")

SOCIOBIOLOGY: THE HUMAN ANIMAL (1977, 16mm film, 3/4" or 1/2" videocassette,
 57 min, col)
 Production: WGBH/BBC
 Distribution: Time-Life Video; $700 for 16mm purchase; $200 for 3/4"
   purchase; $150 for 1/2" purchase; $65 for rental

 Examines some of the ideas of sociobiologists, such as the notion that
 morality and justice are traits rooted in the genetic code. The sociobiologists' belief that behavior is biologically determined may be used
 to better understand fields such as law, economics, and anthropology,
 but may also be used to justify inequality, according to this program.

THE SPIRIT POSESSION OF ALEJANDRO MAMANI (1974, 16mm film, 27 min, col,
 English subtitles)
 Production: Hubert Smith, for the American Universities Field Staff
 Distribution: Filmakers Library; $280 for purchase; $40 for rental

 A cross-cultural perspective on aging and bereavement. Alejandro Mamani,
 an Aymara Indian, is suffering isolation and loneliness at the age of
 eighty-one. He fears that he is possessed by evil spirits, and frustrated
 in his efforts to cure himself of these spirits, he resorts to suicide.
 This film provides a cross-cultural examination of attitudes toward aging,
 psychological disorders, healing, and suicide.

THE STREET (1976, 16mm film, 3/4" videocassette, 10 min, col)
 Production: National Film Board of Canada
 Distribution: National Film Board of Canada; $185 for 16mm purchase;
   $150 for 3/4" purchase; $20 for 16mm or 3/4" rental

 An animated story of a family's experience with a grandmother dying at
 home, as seen through the eyes of her nine-year-old grandson.

SYKES (1974, 16mm film, 13 min, col)
 Production: Deirdre Walsh
 Distribution: Filmakers Library; $293 for purchase; $30 for rental

 This film portrays a blind, elderly man as he moves through his daily
 activities with spirit. He is filmed running errands in his neighbor-
 hood and playing the piano in a local bar.

THE SYNDROME OF ORDINARY GRIEF (1971, 3/4" videocassette, 32 min, col)
    Production: University of Texas Medical Branch at Galveston
    Distribution: Dr. Robert B. White; $150 for purchase; $50 for rental

Presents an interview with a sophomore medical student whose only child
(son, age two) was killed in an auto wreck four weeks previously. The
tape is accompanied by a paper on the manifestation and therapeutic
management of grief that is demonstrated in the program.

TERMINAL ILLNESS (1972, series in 6 parts, 3/4" videocassette, b&w)
    Production: Health Sciences Learning Resources Center, and CCTV Services
      of the University of Washington
    Distribution: University of Washington Press; $1200 for series purchase;
      $225 for single program purchase

In 1972, Dr. Gary E. Leinbach was diagnosed as having an inoperable
adenocarcinoma of the small intestine. Over fifteen hours of conversation with Dr. Leinbach, his wife, other physicians, and members of religious communities were taped during the last months of his life, and
immediately following his death. These tapes have been edited into this
six-part series.

Part 1. INTERVIEWS WITH THE PATIENT (25 min)

    Presents interviews between the patient and his psychiatrist, in which
    Dr. Leinbach's fears, anger, and depression are expressed.

Part 2. THE ROLE OF THE PHYSICIAN (41 min)

    Examines the physician's role in the care of the terminally ill,
    including a discussion of the team approach to patient care.

Part 3. PAIN MANAGEMENT (37 min)

    Dr. Leinbach, his family, and several physicians discuss different
    approaches to pain management.

Part 4. RELIGION AND THE CLERGY (35 min)

    Presents conversations between Dr. Leinbach and several ministers of
    different theological backgrounds.

Part 5 and 6. THE GRIEVING PROCESS (25 and 45 min)

    Interviews between Dr. Leinbach's psychiatrist and Mrs. Leinbach are
    shown in these programs. The interviews extend from before Dr. Leinbach's
    death until twelve months following, and exhibit the evolution of the
    grieving process.

THEOLOGY OF DEATH AND DYING (1978, 3/4" videocassette, 64 min, col)
    Production: Creighton University; Thomas J. Shanahan
    Distribution: Learning Resources Center, Bio-Information Center,
      Creighton University; $11.50 for rental

    A lecture on research done on death and the dying person's feelings.
    Also included is discussion of how people learn to cope with the reality
    of their own death.

THEOLOGY OF SUFFERING, HEALTH AND HEALING - BUDDHISM (1978, 3/4" video-
    cassette, 60 min, col)
    Production: Creighton University; Richard J. Hauser
    Distribution: Learning Resources Center, Bio-Information Center,
      Creighton University; $11.50 for rental

    Examines Buddhist beliefs about helping people cope with suffering.

THEOLOGY OF SUFFERING, HEALTH AND HEALING - EVIL AND THE GOD OF LOVE (1978,
    3/4" videocassette, 60 min, col)
    Production: Creighton University; Richard J. Hauser
    Distribution: Learning Resources Center, Bio-Information Center, Creighton
      University; $11.50 for rental

    This program examines a theoretical view of suffering, and suggests ways
    in which man can use the three approaches of Buddhism, the Old Testament,
    and the New Testament to develop an individual approach to dealing with
    suffering.

THEOLOGY OF SUFFERING, HEALTH AND HEALING - NEW TESTAMENT (1979, 3/4" video-
    cassette, 60 min, col)
    Production: Creighton University; Richard J. Hauser
    Distribution: Learning Resources Center, Bio-Information Center, Creighton
      University; $11.50 for rental

    Examines a New Testament view related to suffering.

THEOLOGY OF SUFFERING, HEALTH AND HEALING - OLD TESTAMENT (1979, 3/4" video-
    cassette, 60 min, col)
    Production: Creighton University; Richard J. Hauser
    Distribution: Learning Resources Center, Bio-Information Center, Creighton
      University; $11.50 for rental

    Examines an Old Testament view related to suffering.

TIME TO COME HOME (1979, 16mm film, 24 min, col)
    Production: University of Minnesota, Department of Physical Medicine and
      Rehabilitation
    Distribution: Department of Physical Medicine and Rehabilitation; $275
      for purchase; $35 for rental

Portrays the home care of dying children. Three families dealing with
home care are shown, and illustrate the value of nurses in these
situations.

TITICUT FOLLIES (1967, 16mm film, 89 min, b&w)
    Production: Frederick Wiseman
    Distribution: Zipporah Films; $1200 for 5-year lease; $150 for
      rental

This film is set in a state mental hospital in Massachusetts. It is a
grim documentary of conditions in this hospital, done in the same manner
as "Hospital." Inmates and staff are seen in recreation, treatment, dis-
cipline, and daily maintenance.

TO AGE IS HUMAN (1975, series in 5 parts, 16mm film, 3/4" videocassette)
    Production: Penn State Television
    Distribution: Pennsylvania State University, Audio Visual Services

This series presents the problems of aging from a number of varying perspectives.

    Part 1. THE FINAL, PROUD DAYS OF ELSIE WURSTER (58 min, b&w)
      Distribution: $315 for 16mm purchase; $205 for 3/4" purchase;
        $16.50 for 16mm rental; $16 for 3/4" rental

      Filmed in a nursing home during the last 44 days of Elsie Wurster's
      life, this program examines her treatment and feelings during the
      period.

    Part 2. THE FACES OF A-WING (58 min, b&w)
      Distribution: $315 for 16mm purchase; $205 for 3/4" purchase;
        $16.50 for 16mm rental; $16 for 3/4" rental

      This program uses vignettes and little narration to illustrate life
      in the "A"-Wing of a nursing home.

    Part 3. MORE THAN A PLACE TO DIE (59 min, b&w)
      Distribution: $205 for 3/4" purchase; $16 for 3/4" rental

      David Reed, administrator of a non-profit nursing home, discusses the
      problems and his philosophy of administering this type of home.

    Part 4. NEVER TOO LATE (58 min, col)
      Distribution: $335 for 3/4" purchase; $22.50 for 3/4" rental

      Presents elderly people from both rural and urban communities discussing
      the problems of old age.

Part 5. OLD MYTHS, NEW REALITIES (58 min, col)
   Distribution: $335 for 3/4" purchase; $22.50 for 3/4" rental

   This program seeks to disrupt stereotypes regarding the aged. Included
   are interviews with James Michener, now in his seventies, and experts in
   gerontology, geriatrics, and social services.

TO DIE TODAY (1970, 16mm film, 3/4" videocassette, 50 min, b&w)
   Production: Canadian Broadcasting Corporation
   Distribution: Filmakers Library; $425 for 16mm purchase; $375 for
   3/4" purchase; $45 for 16mm rental

   Presents an interview with Dr. Elisabeth Kubler-Ross regarding her research
   in stages of acceptance of dying patients. A group discussion is presented
   which focuses on needs of the dying patient for the support of health care
   professionals. Attitudes toward death are explored, as are the patient's
   need for normal interaction, and for acceptance of death as an intrinsic
   part of life.

TO DIE WITH DIGNITY: TO LIVE WITH GRIEF (1978, 3/4" videocassette, 29 min, col)
   Production: Michigan Media
   Distribution: Michigan Media; $25 for rental

   The following individuals discuss their views on coping with death and living
   with grief: a terminally ill leukemia patient, a terminal care physician,
   a minister who counsels health care professionals as well as patients and
   their relatives, and a couple who lose a son.

TO RAISE THE INTELLIGENCE OF THE STATE (1980, audiocassette, 29 min)
   Production: National Public Radio
   Distribution: National Public Radio; $6 for purchase

   Wendy Blair interviews the principals in the Carrie Buck case, which recently
   brought attention to the sterilization laws of the 1920s and 1930s. During
   this period, involuntary eugenic sterilization was permitted for those deemed
   unfit for childbirth, in order to "raise the intelligence of the state." The
   program notes that the Nazi sterilization laws of the 1930s were modeled
   after the 1924 West Virginia Eugenic Sterilization Laws.

THE TOTAL PICTURE
   (see series: "The Family and its Relationship to the Developmentally Disabled: Legal, Ethical, and Moral Issues" - Part 4)

THE ULTIMATE EXPERIMENTAL ANIMAL - MAN (1973, 16mm film, 3/4", 1/2", or 1/4"
   videocassette, 37 min, col)
   Production: National Broadcasting Co.
   Distribution: Films, Inc.; $560 for 16mm purchase; $280 for 3/4", 1/2",
   or 1/4" purchase; $60 for 16mm rental

Examines ethical problems surrounding experimentation with human subjects.
The value of experimentation to medical advancement is discussed, as well
as some abuses of human experimentation.

UNTIL I DIE (1970, 16mm film, 3/4" videocassette, 30 min, col)
   Production: Barey Callari, Gloria Callari
   Distribution: American Journal of Nursing Co. (New York) for purchase;
      American Journal of Nursing Co., Videotape Library (Chicago) for rental;
      $395 for 16mm purchase; $265 for 3/4" purchase; $35 for 16mm rental;
      $30 for 3/4" rental

Presentations of interviews with clinical patients and hospital staff personnel are used in this program on death and dying. Dr. Elisabeth Kubler-
Ross stresses the need for hospital personnel to reach out to help the
dying patient. She describes her theory of the five stages through which
patients with a terminal illness go in order to come to a peaceful acceptance of their imminent death. Patients are shown during each of these stages,
and Dr. Kubler-Ross suggests some hints which might be of help in dealing
with these patients. She stresses honesty in dealing with patients with
terminal illness.

VALLEY OF THE SHADOW: A JOURNEY THROUGH GRIEF (1980, 16mm film, 3/4" video-
   cassette, 38 min, col)
   Production: 20/20 Media
   Distribution: Creative Marketing; $450 for 16mm purchase; $315 for 3/4"
      purchase; $50 for 16mm rental; $40 for 3/4" rental

A couple reflect on the tragic death of their two children. Both the event
itself and its aftermath are discussed. In the latter half of this tape,
experts comment on the father's development of multiple myeloma as a possible biochemical grief reaction.

VALUES CLARIFICATION (1980, slide and audiocassette, 16 min, col)
   Production: Concept Media; Janet Freebairn, Karen Gwinup
   Distribution: Concept Media, $98 for purchase

Outlines the theory of values clarification and the seven steps in the
valuing process. Also discussed in the program are several complex issues
of an ethical nature around which health care professionals need to clarify
their values, according to the producers.

VIEWPOINT: THE DYING PATIENT (1972, filmstrip and audiocassette, 31 min, col,
   guide)
   Production: Concept Media; Karen Gwinup, Shirley A. Carey, Donna C.
      Aguilera
   Distribution: Concept Media; $98 for purchase

Presents pictures of and discussions by two dying patients who describe
their feelings and reactions to the experience.

VIEWPOINT: THE NURSE (1972, filmstrip and audiocassette, 26 min, col, guide)
    Production: Concept Media; Karen Gwinup, Shirley A. Carey, Donna C.
     Aguilera
    Distribution: Concept Media; $98 for purchase

Presents pictures of and discussions by two nurses who describe their
feelings and reactions toward caring for dying patients.

WAITING TO DIE (1980, audiocassette, 29 min)
    Production: National Public Radio
    Distribution: National Public Radio; $6 for purchase

This program suggests that anticipating death does not have to be a de-
pressing experience. Health professionals, ministers, and the elderly talk
about dying, and agree that one need not fear old age. They examine the
attitudes of younger people toward the elderly.

WHEN SHOULD LIFE END? (1979, audiocassette, 59 min)
    Production: National Public Radio
    Distribution: National Public Radio; $7 for purchase

Describes advances in medical technology which have made it possible to
keep the human body alive almost indefinitely. Doctors, patients, and
others present varying opinions about prolonging life, the process of dying
and the avoidance of death.

WHERE IS DEAD? (1976, 16mm film, 3/4" or 1/2" videocassette, 19 min, col)
    Production: Lifestyle Productions
    Distribution: Encyclopedia Brittanica Educational Corporation; $285 for
     16mm, 3/4", or 1/2" purchase; $16 for 16mm, 3/4", or 1/2" rental

An examination of the feelings and process of grief of the parents of a
child who has died in a tragic accident.

WHO SHALL PLAY GOD? (1978, audiocassette, 59 min)
    Production: National Public Radio
    Distribution: National Public Radio; $7 for purchase

Ted Howard, co-author of Who Shall Play God?, discusses genetic engineering.
Focusing on the future social application of this research, he explores the
involvement of government, business and science in promoting genetic engineering. Mr. Howard explores some current uses of this research, and
talks about cloning, artificial insemination, and genetic screening tests
for employment.

WHO SHOULD SURVIVE? (Early 1970s, 16mm, 26 min)
    Production: Joseph P. Kennedy, Jr. Foundation
    Distribution: Lowengard & Brotherhood; $185 for purchase; $25 for rental

A dramatic reenactment of one hospital's decision not to treat a Down's
Syndrome baby with an intestinal blockage. The child needed an operation
to clear an intestinal blockage in order to live, but the parents refused
treatment. The surgeon and the hospital concurred in the parents' decision
not to operate on the intestinal blockage. The baby was put in a side room
and was not fed. After fifteen days it died. The ethical and legal issues
raised by this incident are examined. (This film is sometimes shown with
"A Question of Values.")

WHOSE LIFE IS IT ANYWAY? (1975, 16mm film, 53 min, col)
    Production: Granada TV International
    Distribution: Concern for Dying; $600 for purchase; $60 for rental

Ken Harrison, a thirty-five-year-old sculptor whose spinal cord was damaged
in a road accident, leaving him permanently without the use of his arms or
legs, questions whether life is worth living in his new condition. Issues
include the following: quality of life, informed consent, competency,
patient advocacy, paternalism, sexual identity and self-worth, professional
obligations, and patients' rights. (It is the same story which inspired
the play and commercial film.)

WHY ME? (1978, 3/4" videocassette, 10 min, col)
    Production: National Film Board of Canada; Derek Lamb, Janet Perlman
    Distribution: Pyramid Films; $200 for purchase; $45 for rental

This animated film illustrates an individual's reactions when he learns
he is going to die. Nesbitt Spoon learns he has only five minutes to
live, and undergoes a series of responses representative of typical reactions to terminal illness.

WINNING BATTLES: CHILDREN WITH CANCER (1979, 16mm film 8 min, col)
    Production: Rob Frutchman
    Distribution: Filmakers Library; $250 for purchase; $30 for rental

Dr. Jordan Wilbur of the Children's Cancer Research Institute in San
Francisco is featured in this film about his new program at Stanford
University Children's Hospital. In his program he encourages warm and
open family support of children suffering from cancer. He believes that
the possibility of death should be discussed with the child, but that
hope should be maintained for the future.

WORKING WITH DEATH (1976, series in 3 parts, 16mm film, 3/4" videocassette,
   col, guide)
   Production: The Filmakers
   Distribution: American Video Services; $395 for 16mm or 3/4" series
      purchase; $200 for 16mm or 3/4" single program purchase; $150 for
      16mm or 3/4" series rental: $50 for 16mm or 3/4" single program rental

   Part 1. DEATH AND THE DOCTOR (16 min)

   Portrays the stress upon physicians who treat terminally ill patients.

   Part 2. THE DYING PATIENT (19 min)

   Examines the following topics: terminal care, attitudes toward death,
   truth disclosure, and physician-patient relations.

   Part 3. THE FAMILY (16 min)

   Presents a panel of family support persons discussing the psychological
   needs of families of the dying or the newly dead in coping with bereavement.

YOU SEE, I'VE HAD A LIFE (1972, 16mm film, 32 min, b&w)
   Production: Ben Levin
   Distribution: Vince Books; apply for purchase: $40 for rental

   Portrays a thirteen-year-old boy, Paul Hendricks, who has leukemia. He
   is seen in school, exercising, and in the hospital. Family, friends,
   teachers, and doctors all contribute to the discussion of Paul's life
   and illness.

APPENDIX: PANEL DISCUSSION AND LECTURE SERIES

I. BIOMEDICAL ETHICS (series in 17 parts, 3/4" or 1/2" videocassette, col)
   Production: The University of Texas Health Science Center at Dallas
   Distribution: Mrs. Esther Ruiz; $1,000 for 3/4" or 1/2" series
   purchase; $750 for 3/4" or 1/2" purchase of any 12 programs, $500
   for 3/4" or 1/2" purchase of any 8 programs; $75 for 3/4" or 1/2"
   single program purchase; $30 for 3/4" or 1/2" single program rental.

This series of programs represents an entire course in Biomedical
Ethics taught at the University of Texas.

Part 1. DEATH AND DYING (1977, 50 min)

Ivan Danhof, M.D., Ph.D., presents the experienced physician's viewpoint of many issues involved in this topic. Included in this presentation are comments on the definition of death, the legal problems
of defining death, cross cultural views of death, and conflicting
societal paradoxes involving death.

Part 2. PHILOSOPHICAL BASIS OF BIOMEDICAL ETHICS (1977, 58 min)

Richard Zaner, Ph.D., represents the academic philosophical community's approach to the broad scope of biomedical ethics, stressing
the need to deal with the "whole patient" rather than just the dis-
eased or injured portion. Emphasis is placed on patients' rights
and doctors' responsibilities in the doctor-patient relationship.

Part 3. ETHICAL ISSUES IN HUMAN GENETICS (1977, 55 min)

Mary Jo Harrod, Ph.D., addresses ethical issues in the area of
human genetics. Included in this presentation is coverage of the
following topics: genetic screening, genetic counseling, the
right to privacy of patients' medical records, and genetic engineering.

Part 4. DRUGS, MEDICINE AND THE LAW (1977, 47 min)

Charles Galvin, J.D., discusses a new, positive perspective of
medical-legal relations to offset the bitterness caused by malpractice lawsuits. He emphasizes the cooperative efforts of medicine and law in dealing with issues such as drug abuse, development of new drugs, and the natural death legislation now in effect
in several states.

Part 5. ETHICAL ISSUES IN SERVICE FOR THE AGED (1977, 47 min)

Charles White, Ph.D., analyzes several problems faced by those
persons over sixty-five in our population. These problems are
viewed as they fit into the following ethical concepts:
pateranlism, utilitarianism, egalitarianism, a social contract
formula, and distributive justice.

Part 6. ETHICS OF ORGAN TRANSPLANTATION (1977, 57 min)

Alan Hull, M.D., and Tom Sampson, Ph.D., examine the human non-
technical issues involved in organ transplantation. These ethical considerations include the right of a person to donate an
organ, the use of cadaverous organs in transplants, the cost of
transplants, and the family implications of such operations.

Part 7. GRIEF AS EXPERIENCED BY THE BEREAVED AND THE PATIENT
(1977, 58 min)

Chaplain Herman Cook draws on his hospital experience to teach
a first aid lesson in grieving. He touches on such emotions as
anticipatory grief, hostile reactions, identification with the
deceased, the bargaining process, and the need for good, open
communications.

Part 8. GRIEF AS EXPERIENCED BY THE HELPER SUBJECTIVELY AND
OBJECTIVELY (1977, 44 min)

Chaplain Herman Cook explores the area of the "third grief" as
experienced by all members of the health care team. Stress is
placed on the need to recognize and deal with the multiple psy-
chic wounds physicians and staff might suffer in handling patients,
the special needs of emergency room personnel, and the possibilities of alternative systems of health care, such as hospices.

Part 9. MEDICAL LEGAL ETHICS (1980, 58 min)

Carla Dowben, J.D., outlines the basic problems that have arisen
between the professions of medicine and law. Besides outlining
eight basic steps physicians can use to keep from being sued, Dr.
Dowben also deals with privileged information, informed consent,
negligence, and the rights of minors and the mentally retarded.

Part 10. ETHICS IN PSYCHIATRIC COUNSELING (1977, 59 min)

Barry Rosson, M.D., looks at medical ethics from the psychiatrist's
viewpoint and comes up with several major dilemmas. Besides the
broader topics of confidentiality, informed consent, and cost
effectiveness, he also deals with the more specific subjects of
institutionalizing patients against their will, children involved
in psychiatric treatment, and custodial vs. actual medical care in
today's mental institutions.

Part 11. ETHICS IN HEALTH CARE MANAGEMENT (1977, 52 min)

Ruben Meyer, M.D., examines the broad, societal approaches toward
health care delivery in modern America, dividing the public atti-

tudes into egalitarianism vs. liberatarianism. The main topics
addressed include the cost of health care, consumers' demands for
more health care, and new consumers' perspectives on the "right"
to health care."

Part 12. ETHICS IN THE CARE OF THE MENTALLY RETARDED (1977, 56 min)

Roy Martin, D.Min., presents a humanistic approach to the subject
of the mentally retarded, stressing the situation faced by the
mentally ill child. Particular emphasis is placed on society's
attitudes toward these children, a system of values clarification
that helps the viewer understand these attitudes, and a definition
of what is meant by being "human," as this term regards birth
defectives.

Part 13. PATIENT RESPONSIBILITY IN HEALTH CARE (1980, 47 min)

Jean Achterberg, Ph.D., examines the current status of medicine
in relation to the following major problems: economic, techno-
logical, and humanistic. Stress is placed on the role of behavioral change which allows the individual to improve his or her own
health in areas where traditional medicine has proven ineffective.

Part 14. THE VALUE COMPONENT OF PLANNED PARENTHOOD DECISIONS (1980,
46 min)

Judith Erlen, Ph.D., R.N., presents current options available in
making a planned parenthood decision and examines value factors
which influence this decision. Special emphasis is placed on the
proper roles and the techniques to be used by the health care professional who is facilitating this decision-making process.

Part 15. ETHICAL ISSUES IN THE CARE OF THE HOSPITALIZED CHILD (1980.
59 min)

Sally Francis, M.A., M.S., presents historical background and
relates it to the current problems faced by the hospitalized
child. Special attention is given to effective techniques which
are being used in some hospitals to improve the physical and emotional care of children, from childhood through adolescence.

Part 16. VALUE CONFLICTS IN THE PRACTICE OF HEALTH CARE (1980,
47 min)

Roy Martin, D.Min., examines stresses which exist in the hospital
environment and shows how this pressure can lead to tension between
and ineffectiveness among health care professionals. Extra emphasis
is placed on techniques to lessen this stress and promote collabora-
tive working efforts in hospital settings.

Part 17. BASIS FOR PARTICIPANT RIGHTS IN HEALTH CARE (1980, 53 min)

Ronald Anderson, M.D., traces the historic evolution of the current patient-physician relationship, emphasizing the rights of the patient and the physician's responsibility to uphold these rights. Special attention is placed on the importance of the overall health care team and need to place the patient at the center of medical decision-making.

II. ETHICAL ISSUES IN MEDICINE AND HEALTH CARE (1981, series in 5 parts, 3/4" or 1/2" videocassette, each program 60 min, col)
    Production: Thomas R. McCormick
    Distribution: Thomas R. McCormick; $5 for 3/4" or 1/2" rental
    Host Lecturer: Thomas R. McCormick, D.Min., Department of Bio-
       medical History, School of Medicine, University of Washington

Part 1. ABORTION

Patricia Valdez, Director of Abortion Referral Services, is interviewed. A short lecture by McCormick is included, in which he examines reasons why people seek abortions, ethical theories which may pertain to the decision, and many factors which make abortion a complex dilemma.

Part 2. GENETICS

Eugene Edgar, Ph.D., Professor of Special Education, and affil-iated with the Child Development and Mental Retardation Center is featured. A short lecture by McCormick includes discussion of amniocentesis, genetic screening, uses of genetic information, positive and negative eugenics.

Part 3. WHO SHALL LIVE?

McCormick discusses progress in encouraging life, AID, in vitro fertilization, surrogate mothers, and neonatal intensive care. Case presentation of a premature newborn, and introduction of the Potters Box, a paradigm for ethical decision-making, are included. The dilemma of maximum care vs. palliative care for some cases is also discussed.

Part 4. HUMAN EXPERIMENTATION AND INFORMED CONSENT

Keith and Karlene Trandell-Korenchuk are interviewed. The concept of informed consent, society's concern for the progress of scientific knowledge, the abuses of Nuremberg, and the need for respect and pro-tection of the individual are all discussed. The Potters Box is again presented. The program debates Kant vs. Utilitarianism.

Part 5. DEATH AND DYING

Margy Anderson, Counselor for the School of Medicine, University of Washington, is interviewed. She talks about her personal ex-periences in dealing with a life-threatening cancer. A short lecture by McCormick discusses the history of how people die in America, and a cluster of ethical issues which emerge around dying, including truth-telling, curing vs. caring, and the Natural Death Act.

III. ETHICS AND MEDICINE (1976, series in 11 parts, 3/4" videocassette, each program 60 min, col)
Production: WBGU-TV
Distribution: WBGU-TV for purchase; The Ohio Program in the Humanities for rental; $750 for series purchase; $75 for single program purchase; seven-day free loan
Host: Dr. Thomas Attig, Assistant Professor of Philosophy at Bowling Green State University, Ohio

Part 1. BIO MEDICAL ETHICS: THE RIGHT TO LIVE AND THE RIGHT TO DIE

Interviews with medical and legal professionals and humanists.

Part 2. BIO MEDICAL ETHICS: PROBLEMS OF THE ALLOCATION OF SCARCE LIFE SAVING THERAPY

A lecture presentation by Dr. Richard Wasserstrom, Professor of Philosophy and Professor of Law, University of California at Los Angeles.

Part 3. BIO MEDICAL ETHICS: IS THERE A RIGHT TO DIE?

A lecture presentation by Dr. Wasserstrom.

Part 4. BIO MEDICAL ETHICS: THE DETERMINATION OF DEATH

A lecture presentation by Dr. Wasserstrom.

Part 5. BIO MEDICAL ETHICS: ACTIVE EUTHANASIA

A panel discussion.

Panel: Dr. Marvin Kohl, Professor of Philosophy, State University of New York, College at Fredonia
Karen Metzler, Health Care Consultant, Parma, Ohio
Dr. John Monagle, Director of the Department of Human Values in Medicine, St. Vincent Medical Center, Toledo, Ohio

Part 6. CONFLICTING RIGHTS IN HEALTH CARE: ACCOUNTABILITY: PROBLEMS WITH PSROs AND THE RIGHT TO COMPETENT CARE

An address given by Dr. Robert Veatch, Associate for Medical Ethics for the Institute of Society, Ethics and the Life

Sciences, at Hastings-on-Hudson, New York, with Dr. John Smithson, an internist from Findlay, as reactor.

Part 7. CONFLICTING RIGHTS IN HEALTH CARE: THE RIGHT NOT TO BE A PATIENT

An address given by Dr. Thomas S. Szasz, Professor of Psychiatry, State University of New York at Syracuse, New York, with Dr. Timothy B. Moritz, Director of the Ohio Department of Mental Health and Mental Retardation, as reactor.

Part 8. CONFLICTING RIGHTS IN HEALTH CARE: THE PATIENT'S RIGHT TO KNOW THE TRUTH

An address given by Dr. Judith Swazey, Associate Professor of Socio-Medical Sciences at Boston University School of Medicine, with Dr. David Benson, Assistant Professor of Law, Ohio Northern University, as reactor.

Part 9. CONFLICTING RIGHTS IN HEALTH CARE: SOME PROBLEMS OF DISTRIBUTIVE JUSTICE

An address by Dr. Ronald Benson, Associate Professor of Philosophy, Ohio Northern University, followed by a panel discussion.

Panel: Dr. William Ruse, Administrator, Blanchard Valley Hospital, Findlay
David Rosebrock, Health Commissioner, Combined Allen County (Ohio) General Health District
Dr. Paul Fishman, Physician with Emergency Medical Services, Inc., at Lima Memorial Hospital
Moderator: Louis Vottero, Associate Professor of Pharmacy and Assistant Dean of the College of Pharmacy, Ohio Northern University

Part 10. CONFLICTING RIGHTS IN HEALTH CARE: THE RIGHTS OF REPRODUCTION

An address given by Dr. James R. Sorenson, Associate Professor of Socio-Medical Sciences at Boston University School of Medicine, with Dr. Matthew Suffness, Associate Professor of Pharmacognosy, Ohio Northern University, as reactor.

Part 11. CONFLICTING RIGHTS IN HEALTH CARE: DECISIONS CONCERNING RIGHTS TO LIFE AND DEATH

A lecture presentation by Dr. Daniel Callahan, Director, Institute of Society, Ethics and the Life Sciences, at Hastings-on-Hudson, New York

IV. UNIFORMED SERVICES UNIVERSITY OF THE HEALTH SCIENCES VIDEOTAPES (1978-
    1981, series in 7 parts, 3/4" videocassette, col)
    Production: Uniformed Services University of the Health Sciences,
      School of Medicine
    Distribution: Dr. Edmund G. Howe; $33 for single program purchase;
      free loan

This is a lecture series (listings are alphabetical)

ACTIVE AND PASSIVE EUTHANASIA - ETHICAL CONSIDERATIONS (1979, 60 min)

  Lecturer: James Childress

ETHICAL ASPECTS OF PREVENTIVE MEDICINE (1980, 60 min)

  Lecturer: Ruth Faden

HEALTH CARE - THE CONSUMER'S PERSPECTIVE (1978, 60 min)

  Lecturer: Sidney Wolfe

INFORMED CONSENT - ETHICAL AND LEGAL CONSIDERATIONS (1980, 60 min)

  Lecturer: LeRoy Walters

INTRODUCTION AND CONCLUSION TO BIOETHICS (1978, 4 hrs)

  Lecturer: Samuel Gorovitz

MACROALLOCATION (1979, 60 min)

  Lecturer: Tom Beauchamp

THE PATIENT-PHYSICIAN RELATIONSHIP IN THE MILITARY (1978, 60 min)

  Lecturers: Tris Engelhardt, Bob Joy

V. UCLA MEDICINE AND SOCIETY FORUM VIDEOTAPES (1974-1981, series in 72
   parts, 3/4" videocassette, each program 60 min, b&w unless color is
   indicated)
   Production: UCLA Media Center; Bernard Towers
   Distribution: UCLA Instructional Media Library; $135 for single
     program purchase; $46 for single program rental

This is a panel series, moderated by Bernard Towers, Professor of
Pediatrics and Anatomy, Co-Director, The UCLA Program in Medicine,
Law and Human Values, or by William J. Winslade, Adjunct Professor
of Law and Adjunct Associate Professor of Psychiatry, Co-Director,
The UCLA Program in Medicine, Law and Human Values (listings are
alphabetical.)

ABORTION: IS THERE STILL AN ETHICAL PROBLEM? (12/75)

Panel: Irvin M. Cushner, Associate Professor of Obstetrics &
        Gynecology and Public Health
       William J. Dignam, Professor of Obstetrics & Gynecology
       Rachel Pape, Assistant Clinical Professor of Psychiatry
       Richard A. Wasserstrom, Professor of Law & Philosophy

ASSISTED SUICIDE: IS IT ALWAYS WRONG? (3/79)

Panel: Derek Humphry, Journalist
       Arthur Rosett, Professor of Law
       Joel Yager, Associate Professor of Psychiatry

ATTEMPTED SUICIDE: WHAT CONSTITUTES APPROPRIATE MEDICAL CARE?
(6/74)

Panel: James Brill, Director, Hospital Emergency Service
       Daniel H. Simmons, Professor of Medicine and
         Physiology
       L. Jolyon West, Professor and Chairman, Department
         of Psychiatry
       Daniel I. Wikler, Teaching Fellow, Department of
         Philosophy

BABIES WITH SHORT-BOWEL SYNDROME: IS VIGOROUS THERAPY ALWAYS
APPROPRIATE? (5/79)

Panel: Marvin Ament, Professor of Pediatrics/Gastroenterology
       Eric Fonkalsrud, Professor of Surgery
       James Read, Teaching Fellow, Dept. of Philosophy

THE BATTERED CHILD SYNDROME (2/75)

Panel: Frank R. Ervin, Professor of Psychiatry
       L. Robert Martin, Professor of Medicine/Family Practice
       Richard A. Wasserstrom, Professor of Law & Philosophy

BEHAVIOR MODIFICATION: TREATMENT OR COERCION? (6/75)

Panel: James Q. Simmons, III, Associate Professor of
         Psychiatry
       Daniel I. Wikler, Teaching Fellow, Department of
         Philosophy
       Lynn Wikler, Associate in Psychiatry

BLOOD FOR TRANSFUSION: TO GIVE OR TO TRADE? (2/77)

Panel: Robert Adams, Professor of Philosophy
       Norman R. Kear, Administrator of L.A./Orange Counties
         Red Cross Program
       Byron A. Myhre, Professor of Pathology; Vice-President,
         American Association of Blood Banks

BONE-MARROW TRANSPLANTATION: THERAPY OR EXPERIMENT?
PART I: CLINICAL ASPECTS (5/76)

   Panel: Stephen A. Feig, Assistant Professor of Pediatrics/
           Hematology
        Robert P. Gale, Assistant Professor of Medicine &
           Medical Microbiology
        William N. Valentine, Professor of Medicine/Hematology

BONE-MARROW TRANSPLANATION: THERAPY OR EXPERIMENT?
PART II: SOCIETAL, ETHICAL AND PSYCHOLOGICAL ASPECTS (3/77)

   Panel: Philippa Foot, Professor of Philosophy
        Renee C. Fox, Professor and Chairman, Department
           of Sociology and Professor, School of Medicine,
           University of Pennsylvania
        Louis Jolyon West, Professor and Chairman, Depart-
           ment of Psychiatry and Biobehavioral Sciences

BRAIN BIOPSIES IN CHILDREN: WHEN ARE THEY ETHICAL? (3/74)

   Panel: John H. Menkes, Clinical Professor of Pediatrics/
           Neurology
        W. Eugene Stern, Professor of Surgery (Neurosurgery)
        Daniel I. Wikler, Teaching Fellow, Department of
           Philosophy

CALIFORNIA'S NATURAL DEATH ACT: WHAT DIFFERENCE HAS IT MADE? (1/78)

   Panel: M. Steven Lipton, Attorney at Law
        Edwin S. Shneidman, Professor of Thanatology
        William J. Winslade, Lecturer in Law and Psychiatry

CAN HEART DISEASE BE ERADICATED? (2/79)

   Panel: R. James Barnard, Research Cardiologist
        Albert M. Kattus, Professor of Medicine/Cardiology
        Nathan Pritikin, Director, Longevity Center, Santa
           Monica

CANCER AND MARIJUANA: MEDICINE AND THE LAW (10/79)

   Panel: Kenneth W. Graham, Professor of Law
        J. Thomas Ungerleider, Associate Professor of Psychiatry
        Fran Wiley, Clinical Nurse Specialist

CHILD ABUSE AND THE LAW: SERIOUS PROBLEMS AND REAL POSSIBILITIES
(10/80, col)

   Panel: Paul Boland, Professor of Law & Associate Dean
        Morris J. Paulson, Professor of Psychiatry
        Mary J. Spencer, Assistant Professor of Pediatrisc;
           Director, Marion Davies Children's Clinic & Chair-
           man, UCLA SCAN Team

CHILDREN'S RIGHTS: CAN A PHYSICIAN BE A TRUE ADVOCATE? (10/77)

Panel: Michael S. Goldstein, Assistant Professor of Public
           Health and Sociology
         Jacquelyn K. Green, Assistant Professor of Psychiatry
         Mary Ann Lewis, Assistant Professor of Nursing and
           Medicine

DNA RESEARCH AND THE LAW: CO-OPERATION OR COLLISION? (5/77)

Panel: Marc A. Lappe, Chief, Office of Health, Law and Human
           Values, California State Department of Health
         Gary L. Wilcox, Assistant Professor of Bacteriology
         William J. Winslade, Lecturer in Law and Psychiatry

DIALYSING THE ELDERLY: WHO DECIDES AND ON WHAT GROUNDS? (9/80, col)

Panel: Thomas E. Hill, Associate Professor of Philosophy
         Robert L. Kane, Associate Professor of Philosophy
         Barbara Rever, Assistant Professor of Medicine/
           Nephrology

DOWN'S SYNDROME WITH LIFE-THREATENING COMPLICATIONS: WHAT
SHOULD BE DONE? (1/80)

Panel: Dale Phelps, Assistant Professor of Pediatrics/
           Neonatology
         Catherine Sammons, Clinical Social Worker, Clinical
           Research Center for the Study of Childhood Psychosis;
           Lecturer in Psychiatry and Biobehavioral Sciences
         William J. Winslade, Lecturer in Law and Psychiatry

EMERGENCY OBSTETRICS: PATIENT RIGHTS AND PHYSICIAN RESPONSIBILITIES
(10/78)

Panel: Sharon Bishop, Professor of Philosophy, Cal State,
           Los Angeles
         Charles R. Brinkman III, Professor of Obstetrics
         Erwin Deutsch, Professor of Law, Univ. of Gottingen,
           Germany

ENERGY NEEDS, RESOURCES AND HEALTH RISKS (1/79)

Panel: Edward L. Alpen, Director, Donner Laboratory of
           Medical Physics, U.C. Berkeley
         Norman Cousins, Senior Lecturer in Medical Humanities
         Russell R. O'Neill, Dean, School of Engineering

ENVIRONMENTAL CARCINOGENS: THE ETHICS AND ECONOMICS OF RESPON-
SIBILITY (6/78)

  Panel: Larry Agran, Instructor in Health and Specialist in
          Environmental Health Legislation
         Charles Heidelberger, Director of Basic Research, USC
         Cancer Institute
         Murray Jarvik, Professor of Psychiatry
         Elizabeth Stern, Professor of Epidemiology

EUTHANASIA: THE PROS AND CONS (5/75)

  Panel: Philippa Foot, Professor of Philosophy
         Charles M. Haskell, Assistant Professor of Medicine
         & Surgery/Oncology
         Herbert Morris, Professor of Law & Philosophy

GENETIC SCREENING: THE PROS AND CONS (9/78)

  Panel: Barbara F. Crandall, Associate Professor of Pediatrics/
         Genetics
         Michael Kaback, Professor of Pediatrics/Genetics
         James E. Read, Teaching Fellow, Dept. of Philosophy

GENITAL HERPES AND ITS TREATMENT: SCIENCE AND ART IN MEDICINE
(1/81, col)

  Panel: Stanley M. Bierman, Associate Clinical Professor of
         Medicine
         Yvonne Bryson, Assistant Professor of Pediatrics/
         Infectious Diseases
         Susan C. M. Scrimshaw, Associate Professor of Public
         Health

HEALTH CARE QUALITY ASSURANCE PROGRAMS: HOW EFFECTIVE ARE THEY?
(4/77)

  Panel: Linda K. Demlo, Senior Professional Associate, Insti-
         tute of Medicine, Washington, DC
         John R. Gamble, Professor and Chairman, Department of
         Medicine, Pacific Medical Center, San Francisco
         Charles E. Lewis, Professor of Medicine, Public
         Health and Nursing
         Paul H. Ward, Professor of Surgery/Head and Neck
         Surgery

HOLISTIC MEDICINE AND CONVENTIONAL THERAPY: CONSONANCE OR
DISSONANCE? (4/80, col)

  Panel: David Bresler, Assistant Professor of Anesthesiology;
         Director, Pain Control Unit
         Norman Cousins, Senior Lecturer in Medical Humanities

Jonathan Fielding, Professor of Pediatrics & Public
Health; Co-Director, Center for Health Enhancement
Education and Research

HOW DO ETHICS COMMITTEES DECIDE BETWEEN RIGHT AND WRONG IN CLINICAL
RESEARCH? (3/81, col)

Panel: Albert A. Barber, Vice-Chancellor, Research Programs
Dale Phelps, Assistant Professor of Pediatrics/Neon-
atology
Daniel Wikler, Associate Professor, U. of Wisconsin;
Staff Philosopher, President's Commission for the
Study of Ethical Problems in Medicine, Washington, DC

HOW DOES/SHOULD THE PROSPECT OF DEATH AFFECT OUR LIFE? (9/77)

Panel: Herman Feifel, Chief Psychologist, Veterans Administration Outpatient Clinic, Los Angeles
Philippa Foot, Professor of Philosophy

IF GENETIC SUSCEPTIBILITY TO CANCER IS PREDICTABLE, WHO HAS THE
RIGHT TO KNOW? (9/81, col)

Panel: Eleanor Shur Freidin, Attorney at Law, Retired; former
Counsel, Gateways Hospital and Mental Health Center,
Los Angeles
Richard Gatti, Visiting Professor, Department of Pathology
Jean Hampton, Assistant Professor of Philosophy
Michael B. Van Scoy-Mosher, Clinical Assistant Professor
of Medicine/Oncology, USC Cancer Center; Attending
Physician, Cedars-Sinai Medical Center

THE IMAGE OF THE DOCTOR: HOW AND WHY DO THE MEDIA DISTORT? (2/76)

Panel: Robert F. Epstein, Lecturer in Theater Arts
Christopher Morgan, Producer of Medical Story,
Columbia TV
Karlis Ullis, Associate Physician, Student Health
Service

IMPAIRED MENTAL COMPETENCE IN THE ELDERLY: CHANGES IN THE PATIENT/
PHYSICIAN RELATIONSHIP (2/81, col)

Panel: John C. Beck, Chief of Medicine/Geriatrics
Andrew L. Jameton, Adjunct Assistant Professor,
Health Policy Program, UCSF
Howard F. Wallach, Associate Clinical Professor of
Psychiatry; Chief of Gero-Psychiatry, Sepulveda
V.A. Hospital
Christine K. Cassel, Fellow in Gerontology, V.A.
Hospital, Portland, Oregon

INFORMED CONSENT: IS IT POSSIBLE OR EVEN ALWAYS DESIRABLE? (12/74)

Panel: Joshua S. Golden, Associate Professor of Psychiatry
Leo D. Lagasse, Associate Professor of Obstetrics &
Gynecology
Jeremy H. Thompson, Professor of Pharmacology

INTRAUTERINE DIAGNOSIS IN EARLY PREGNANCY: FETAL, PARENTAL AND
SOCIETAL CONSIDERATIONS (11/74)

Panel: Barbara F. Crandall, Assistant Professor of Pediatrics/
Genetics
Michael M. Kaback, Associate Professor of Pediatrics/
Genetics
Daniel I. Wikler, Teaching Fellow, Department of
Philosophy

IS IT RIGHT TO PRESCRIBE STIMULANT DRUGS FOR HYPERACTIVE CHILDREN
WITH LEARNING PROBLEMS? (9/74)

Panel: Madeline C. Hunter, Principal, University Elementary
School
Leon Oettinger, Jr., Associate Clinical Professor of
Pediatrics
Richard J. Schain, Professor of Pediatrics, Neurology &
Psychiatry

IS THE HOME A GOOD PLACE FOR A BABY TO BE BORN? (6/77)

Panel: Cynthia T. Barrett, Assistant Professor of Pediatrics/
Neonatology
Irvin M. Cushner, Professor of Obstetrics and Gynecol-
ogy and Public Health
Susan Scrimshaw, Assistant Professor of Public Health/
Anthropology

KIDNEY FAILURE AND HEMODIALYSIS: SHOULD EVERYONE BE TREATED? (10/74)

Panel: Ralph Goldman, Professor of Medicine/Nephrology
Jennifer Sandoval, Charge Nurse, Dialysis Unit
Raymond Schultze, Professor of Medicine/Nephrology
Daniel I. Wikler, Teaching Fellow, Department of
Philosophy

LABORATORY EXPERIMENTS IN MEDICAL RESEARCH: ANIMAL RIGHTS AND
HUMAN RESPONSIBILITIES (12/77)

Panel: Josiah Brown, Professor of Medicine
Warren S. Quinn, Associate Professor of Philosophy
Donald O. Walter, Associate Professor of Psychiatry

LAETRILE: THE MEDICAL, MORAL AND LEGAL CONTROVERSY (2/78)

    Panel: Raymond J. Neutra, Associate Professor of Public Health
           Joseph F. Ross, Professor of Medicine
           Don G. Rushing, UCLA Law Student

LIFE-SUPPORT FOR THE NEWBORN: IS IT EVER RIGHT TO STOP? (1/76)

    Panel: Cynthia T. Barrett, Assistant Professor of Pediatrics/
           Neonatology
           George P. Fletcher, Professor of Law
           Albert R. Jonsen, Associate Professor of Bioethics,
           UC San Francisco

MEDICAL CARE IN TERMINAL ILLNESS: WHO SPEAKS FOR THE MENTALLY
RETARDED? (12/78)

    Panel: Carole E. Goldberg, Professor of Law
           Frederick Redlich, Professor of Psychiatry
           Leslie S. Rothenberg, Attorney at Law
           James D. Woolery, Chief Resident, Consultation-
           Liaison Psychiatry

MEDICAL-LEGAL PROBLEMS OF INFORMED CONSENT (10/75)

    Panel: Lou Ashe, Attorney at Law
           Ronald Katz, Professor and Chairman, Department of
           anesthesiology

MILD MENTAL RETARDATION: WHAT RIGHTS, WHAT RESPONSIBILITIES?
(11/75)

    Panel: Linda Andron, Psychiatric Social Worker, Mental Retar-
           dation Program
           Robert Edgerton, Professor of Anthropology, Mental
           Retardation Program
           George Tarjan, Professor of Psychiatry, Mental
           Retardation Program

MILK FORMULA FOR INFANTS: BLESSING OR CURSE? (11/78)

    Panel: Fred E. Case, Professor of Urban Land Economics
           The Reverend Richard W. Gillett, Director, Social
           Concerns Ministry, Pasadena
           Derrick B. Jelliffe, Professor of Pediatrics & Public
           Health

MUST SCIENTIFIC MEDICINE BE IMPERSONAL IN ORDER TO ACHIEVE
EXCELLENCE? (6/76)

    Panel: Rodney Bluestone, Professor of Medicine/Rheumatology
           Sheldon Greenfield, Assistant Professor of Medicine &
           Preventive & Social Medicine

Lowell S. Young, Associate Professor of Medicine/
Infectious Diseases

MUST WE REDEFINE DEATH? (2/74)

Panel: Jesse J. Dukeminier, Jr., Professor of Law
        Morton L. Pearce, Professor of Medicine/Cardiology
        Cynthia C. Scalzi, Clinical Specialist, School of
        Nursing

THE NUCLEAR POWER-PLANT: THREAT OR PROMISE? (4/76)

Panel: John Goldsmith, Epidemiological Studies Department,
        California State Health Department
        J. Morgan Jones, Associate Professor of Operations
        Research, Graduate School of Management
        William E. Kastenberg, Associate Professor of Engineer-
        ing and Applied Science

NURSING HOMES: DO WE NEED THEM? CAN WE HELP THEM? (6/79)

Panel: Julian Feingold, Director, Palm Crest House, Long Beach
        Robert L. Kane, Associate, Professor of Medicine
        Judith K. Miller, Director, National Health Policy
        Forum, George Washington University

PAIN AND ITS RELIEF: EXPECTATIONS, MYTHS AND REALITIES (12/76)

Panel: David Bresler, Adjunct Assistant Professor of Anesthes-
        iology; Director, Pain Control Unit
        Jascha Kessler, Professor of English
        Richard D. Walter, Professor and Chairman, Department
        of Neurology

PREVENTION OR CURE: DO MEDICAL SCHOOLS HAVE THE RIGHT PRIORITIES?
(4/75)

Guest Moderator: Forrest H. Adams, Professor of Pediatrics/
        Cardiology
Panel: Lester Breslow, Dean, School of Public Health, Presi-
        dent, Association of Schools of Public Health
        Sherman M. Mellinkoff, Dean, School of Medicine; Chair-
        man, American Association of Medical Colleges

PRIVATE RIGHTS AND PUBLIC HEALTH (5/74)

Panel: Norman Abrams, Professor of Law
        Lester Breslow, Dean, School of Public Health

PSYCHOPOLITICS: SHOULD MENTAL HEALTH PROFESSIONALS MONITOR THE
BEHAVIOR OF POLITICAL LEADERS? (11/79, col)

Panel: Tom Bates, California State Assemblyman, 12th District
        Milton Greenblatt, Director, NPI Hospital & Clinics;
        Professor and Executive Vice-Chairman, Department
        of Psychiatry and Biobehavioral Sciences

RANDOMIZED CLINICAL TRIALS: RESEARCH DESIGN AND ETHICS OF CONSENT
(5/80, col)

Panel: Robert H. Brook, Associate Professor of Medicine and
        Public Health
        Frances Pizzulli, Attorney at Law
        James D. Woolery, Robert Wood Johnson Veterans
        Administration Clinical Scholar

RESPONSIBILITY FOR INFORMED CONSENT: HOW FAR MUST THE PHYSICIAN GO?
(11/80, col)

Panel: N. Jan Almquist Farmer, Law Student III
        Myron Greengold, Director, Family Practice Residency
        Program, Northridge Hospital Foundation Medical
        Center
        Richard J. Steckel, Director, The UCLA Jonsson Compre-
        hensive Cancer Center & Professor of Radiological
        Sciences and of Radiation Oncology

RISK-TAKING IN MEDICINE: WHAT IS PERMISSIBLE? (9/76)

Panel: Ulrich Batzdorf, Associate Professor of Surgery/
        Neurosurgery
        Thomas E. Hill, Jr., Associate Professor of
        Philosophy
        Ronald L. Katz, Professor and Chairman of
        Anesthesiology

SEX-CHANGE TREATMENT: MEDICAL AND SOCIAL ASPECTS (3/75)

Panel: Willard E. Goodwin, Professor of Surgery/Urology
        Gerald D. Leve, Assistant Clinical Professor of Medicine
        Robert J. Stoller, Professor of Psychiatry

SHOULD THE MENTALLY RETARDED BE ALLOWED TO PROCREATE? (3/80, col)

Panel: Linda Andron, Clinical Social Worker; Lecturer in
        Psychiatry and Biobehavioral Sciences
        Alan F. Charles, Vice-Chancellor for Public Affairs
        Irvin M. Cushner, Professor of Obstetrics & Public
        Health; Deputy Assistant Secretary for Population
        Affairs, DHEW

SPERM BANKS: MEDICAL, ETHICAL AND SOCIAL ASPECTS (4/81, col)

Panel: Barbara Crandall, Associate Professor of Psychiatry &
          Pediatrics
        Jean Hampton, Assistant Professor of Philosophy
        Cappy Miles Rothman, Clinical Instructor, Division
          of Urology; Director, The Southern California
          Cryobank

SPINA BIFIDA WITH MENINGOMYELOCELE: SHOULD WE OPERATE? (1/74)

Panel: Paul H. Crandall, Professor of Surgery (Neurosurgery) &
          Neurology
        Thomas H. Hunter, Professor of Medicine, University of
          Virginia
        Daniel I. Wikler, Teaching Fellow, Department of
          Philosophy

STERILIZATION BEFORE REPRODUCTION: THE RIGHT TO CHOOSE (1/75)

Panel: Irvin M. Cushner, Associate Professor of Obstetrics &
          Gynecology
        J. George Moore, Professor and Chairman, Department of
          Obstetrics & Gynecology
        Robert O. Pasnau, Associate Professor of Psychiatry

STRESS AND SUICIDE: ARE PHYSICIANS AT SPECIAL RISK? (10/79, col)

Panel: Josiah Brown, Professor of Medicine
        Fred Loya, Assistant Professor of Psychiatry
        Gary Nye, Psychiatrist Member, CMA Committee on
          the Well-Being of Physicians

SURROGATE MOTHERS: PRIVATE RIGHT OR PUBLIC WRONG (5/81, col)

Panel: Grace G. Blumberg, Professor of Law
        Ann Garry, Associate Professor of Philosophy, Cal
          State, Los Angeles
        Doryann M. Lebe, Associate Professor of Psychiatry

THERAPEUTIC TRIALS: THE ETHICS OF CLINICAL EXPERIMENTATION (9/75)

Panel: Thomas E. Hill, Associate Professor of Philosophy
        Harold Paulus, Associate Professor of Medicine
        Jeremy H. Thompson, Professor of Pharmacology and
          Chairman, Human Subject Protection Committee

THREATS OF VIOLENCE: THE PSYCHOTHERAPIST'S DILEMMA (3/76)

Panel: Hon. Warren Ferguson, Judge, U.S. District Court
        Paul F. Slawson, Associate Professor of Psychiatry
        William J. Winslade, Lecturer in Law & Psychiatry

TO WHOM DOES/SHOULD THE PATIENT'S CHART BELONG? (10/76)

    Panel: Lucy Eisenberg, Attorney at Law
              Charles E. Lewis, Professor of Medicine & Public Health
              Jeremy H. Thompson, Professor of Pharmacology; Chairman,
                 Human Subjects Protection Committee

THE USE OF PLACEBOS: IS THERE A CONFLICT BETWEEN EFFICACY AND
ETHICS? (5/78)

    Panel: Rogers Albritton, Professor of Philosophy
              Norman Cousins, Editor, The Saturday Review
              Sherman M. Mellinkoff, Dean, School of Medicine

WHAT SHOULD BE THE ROLE OF THE PSYCHIATRIST IN THE CRIMINAL COURT?
(11/76)

    Panel: Robert O. Pasnau, Associate Professor of Psychiatry
              Murray L. Schwartz, Professor of Law
              Louis Jolyon West, Professor and Chairman, Depart-
                 ment of Psychiatry and Biobehavioral Sciences

WHEN MEDICAL EQUIPMENT FAILS, WHO IS RESPONSIBLE? (11/77)

    Panel: Thelma Estrin, Director, Data Processing Laboratory
                 Brain Research Institute
              Richard J. Johns, Professor of Biomedical Engineering,
                 John Hopkins Hospital
              Robert W. Rand, Professor of Neurological Surgery

WHY FERTILIZE HUMAN EGGS IN THE LABORATORY? WHY NOT? (4/79)

    Panel: David Meldrum, Assistant Professor of Obstetrics &
                 Gynecology
              Pierre Soupart, Professor of Obstetrics & Gynecology,
                 Vanderbilt University
              Warren Quinn, Associate Professor of Philosophy

WOMEN AND MEDICAL SCHOOL: WHY SO FEW ON FACULTY? DOES IT REALLY
MATTER, AND IF SO, TO WHOM? (4/78)

    Panel: Jennifer S. Buchwald, Professor of Physiology
              John Garcia, Professor of Psychology and
                 Psychiatry
              Sherna Madan, Medical Student & Ph.D. Candidate in
                 Biochemistry
              Carol M. Newton, Professor of Biomathematics &
                 Radiological Sciences

WOMEN M.D.'s: SPECIAL PROBLEMS? SPECIAL NEEDS? SPECIAL
CONTRIBUTIONS? (2/80, col)

    Panel: Christina Benson, Robert Wood Johnson Clinical Scholar
          in Psychiatry
          Selma Calmes, Assistant Professor of Anesthesiology
          Joel Yager, Associate Professor of Psychiatry

WOULD IT HAVE BEEN ETHICAL TO GIVE SWINE-FLU VACCINE TO CHILDREN
WITHOUT PRIOR TESTING? (1/77)

    Panel: Kenneth M. Boyer, Fellow in Pediatrics/Infectious
          Diseases
          James D. Cherry, Professor of Pediatrics/Infectious
          Diseases
          William J. Winslade, Lecturer in Law and Psychiatry

WOULD YOU LET A NURSE PRACTITIONER OR PHYSICIAN'S ASSISTANT TAKE
CARE OF YOUR BEST FRIEND? (4/74)

    Panel: Rheba De Tornyay, Dean, School of Nursing
          Ralph Goldman, Assistant Dean, Allied Health Sciences
          Raymond M. Kivel, Director, MEDEX, Drew Medical School

VI. UNIVERSITY OF VIRGINIA MEDICAL CENTER VIDEOTAPES (1973-1981, series in
44 parts, 3/4" videocassette, each program 60 min, b&w unless col is
indicated)
Production: University of Virginia Medical Center
Distribution: University of Virginia School of Medicine, The Claude
Moore Health Sciences Library; $24 for single program rental (out-
of-state); $19 for single program rental (Virginia)

This is a series of panel discussion tapes from the University of
Virginia's Medical Center Hours,or Medicine and Society Conferences
(listings are alphabetical).

AUTHORITY AND OBEDIENCE (9/80)

    Oscar A. Thorup, Stephen Worchel, James Childress

IS BEHAVIORAL GENETICS TABOO? THE NEO-LYSENKOISM (10/76)

    Thomas H. Hunter, Bernard D. Davis, Joseph Fletcher

BETWEEN DOCTOR AND PATIENT: HOW INFORMED MUST CONSENT BE? (5/76)

    Browning P. Hoffman

CHILDREN'S RIGHTS AND PARENTAL AUTHORITY (4/79)

   Thomas H. Hunter

COMMUNICATION BETWEEN DOCTORS AND PATIENTS: WHY DON'T WE DO MORE
LISTENING? (3/81, col)

   Thomas H. Hunter

DILEMMAS OF CLINICAL TRIALS (10/73)

   Thomas H. Hunter, Robert Marston, Joseph Fletcher

DISCIPLINARY PROCEDURES IN THE MEDICAL PROFESSION: CAN WE POLICE
OURSELVES? (1976)

   Browning P. Hoffman

ETHICAL PROBLEMS IN CLINICAL TRAINING: WHO LOOKS AFTER THE
PATIENT? (1/81, col)

   Thomas H. Hunter

FETAL RESEARCH (2/76)

   Thomas H. Hunter

THE FORBIDDEN EXPERIMENT (3/75)

   Thomas H. Hunter

GENETICALLY TRANSMITTED DISEASE (9/77)

   Oscar A. Thorup

HAS THE PHYSICIAN THE RIGHT TO STRIKE? (11/75)

   Thomas H. Hunter

THE HEALTH OF PUBLIC FIGURES: WHAT SHOULD BE DISCLOSED? (1/74)

   Thomas H. Hunter

HEART TRANSPLANTS: PROS AND CONS (9/80)

   Thomas H. Hunter

HOSPICE IN THE GENERAL HOSPITAL (9/79)

   Oscar A. Thorup

THE HOSPICE MOVEMENT (10/79)

  Oscar A. Thorup, Cicely Saunders, Carleton Sweetser

HOW DOES ONE DETERMINE ACCEPTABLE RISKS? (12/76)

  Thomas H. Hunter, Richard Wenzel, Joseph Fletcher

HOW FAR SHOULD WE GO? ETHICAL DECISIONS ON THE MEDICAL WARDS (1/79)

  Oscar A. Thorup

HUMAN SPERM BANKS (10/80, col)

  Thomas H. Hunter

THE IMPACT OF INSTITUTIONAL REVIEW BOARDS ON RESEARCH (12/79)

  Thomas H. Hunter

IN VITRO FERTILIZATION (1/79)

  Oscar A. Thorup

INVOLUNTARY CONFINEMENT (2/75)

  Thomas H. Hunter

THE ISOLATED IMMUNE-DEFICIENT INFANT: WHAT ABOUT THE FUTURE?

  Joseph Fletcher, Raphael Wilson, L. Owen Hendley

LAETRILE: THE RIGHT TO CHOOSE (9/77)

  Oscar A. Thorup

THE MEDICAL DEVICES EXPLOSION - WHO PROTECTS THE PATIENT? (11/78)

  Anthony Shaw

MEDICINE AND THE PRESS (4/78)

  Oscar A. Thorup

NURSES AND DOCTORS, CONFLICT OR COOPERATION? (2/79)

  Leslie E. Rudolf

PATIENTS' RIGHTS IN SCREENING FOR GENETIC DEFECTS (1/75)

  Thomas H. Hunter

THE PHYSICIAN AS DOUBLE AGENT (1/77, col)

   Thomas H. Hunter

PRIVACY AND THE COMPUTER: EVERYTHING YOU KNOW ABOUT YOURSELF
BUT HOPED THEY'D NEVER FIND OUT (2/78)

   Oscar A. Thorup

PROBLEMS OF SURROGATE PARENTING (2/81, col)

   Oscar A. Thorup, Walter J. Waddington, James F. Childress

QUALITY OF MEDICAL CARE: MEDICINE'S ACCOUNTABILITY TO SOCIETY -
IS PEER REVIEW THE ANSWER? (12/74)

   Thomas H. Hunter

RECOMBINANT DNA RESEARCH AND THE WORLD OF BUSINESS (10/80)

   Thomas H. Hunter

RESEARCH USING "LIVE" HUMAN FETUSES: WHEN IS IT JUSTIFIED? (4/74)

   Thomas H. Hunter

SHOULD WE ALLOW JUDGES TO MAKE MEDICAL DECISIONS? (12/78)

   Thomas H. Hunter

SHOULD WE LEGALIZE THE LIVING WILL? (9/75)

   Thomas H. Hunter

SHOULD YOU CHOOSE YOUR BABY'S SEX: AMNIOCENTESIS FOR SEX
SELECTION (9/80)

   Thomas H. Hunter

SOCIOBIOLOGY: ARE THERE AREAS OF FORBIDDEN KNOWLEDGE? (3/78)

   Oscar A. Thorup

STATISTICAL MORALITY: THE PRICE OF HUMAN LIFE (11/77)

   Oscar A. Thorup

STAY OF EXECUTION: WHEN SHOULD WE TREAT INFECTIONS IN DYING
PATIENTS? (2/74)

   Thomas H. Hunter

TO SAVE OR LET DIE? THE INFANT WITH MYELOMENINGOCELE (4/75)

   Robert M. Blizzard

WHAT RIGHTS DO PATIENTS HAVE? (12/73)

   Thomas H. Hunter

WHO PROTECTS THE VICTIM?   MEDICAL CONFIDENTIALITY (10/75)

   Thomas H. Hunter

YOUR MEDICAL RECORD: HOW CONFIDENTIAL IS IT? (3/79)

   Thomas H. Hunter

TOPICAL INDEX

AGING

Video

The Challenges of Aging: Change
  and Loss, 6
Chillysmith Farm, 6
The Faces of A-Wing, 42
The Final, Proud Days of Elsie
  Wurster, 42
The Geriatric Patient, 19
Growing Old in America, 19
Miss Larsen: Rebel at 90, 27
More Than a Place to Die, 42
Never Too Late, 42
Old Myths, New Realities, 43
Passing Quietly Through, 30
Peege, 30
Secrets, 38
The Spirit Possession of Alejandro
  Mamani, 39
The Street, 39
Sykes, 39

Panel Discussion and Lecture

Dialysing the Elderly: Who
  Decides and on What Grounds?,
  58
Ethical Issues in Service for
  the Aged, 49
Impaired Mental Competence in
  the Elderly: Changes in the
  Patient/Physician Relation-
  ship, 60
Nursing Homes: Do We Need
  Them? Can We Help Them?,
  63

Audio

Aging: Exploring the Myths, 2
The Other Generation Gap, 29

DEATH AND DYING

Video

An Adolescent Copes with
  Cancer, 2
And We Were Sad, Remember?, 2
Attitudes Toward Death and
  Dying, 3
A Conversation with a Widow, 6
Dead Birds, 8
Death, 8
Death and Dying, 20
Death and the Doctor, 47
Death of a Gandy Dancer, 9
The Death of a Newborn, 9
Detour, 10
A Dose of Reality, 11
Dreamspeaker, 12
Dying, 12
The Dying Patient, 47
Elegy, 12
Facing Death, 7
The Family, 47
A Family Copes with Malignant
  Uncertainty, 16
The Father, 16
Finances/Insurance, 7
Fritzi: Living and Dying with
  Dignity, 17
From Both Ends of the Stethescope,
  17
Grief Therapy, 19
The Grieving Process, 40
Hospice, 21
Hospice Encounters and Mental
  Health Training Film, 21
How Could I Not Be among You?,
  22
Interviews with the Patient, 40
Joan Robinson: One Woman's Story,
  24
Jocelyn, 24

Panel Discussion and Lecture

Audio

ETHICS IN HEALTH CARE AND SCIENTIFIC RESEARCH (General)

Video

Audio

GENETICS

Video

Panel Discussion and Lecture

HEALTH CARE PROFESSIONAL/ PATIENT RELATIONSHIP

Video

Panel Discussion and Lecture

HUMAN EXPERIMENTATION AND INFORMED CONSENT

Video

Panel Discussion and Lecture

DISTRIBUTORS

American Humanist Association
Attention: Pat Pliss
7 Horwood Drive
Amherst, NY 14226
tel: 716/839-5080

American Journal of Nursing Co.
555 West 57th Street
New York, NY 10019
tel: 212/582-8820

American Journal of Nursing Co.
Videotape Library
205 West Wacker Drive - Suite 300
Chicago, IL 60606
tel: 312/828-1146

American Video Services
1930 Century Park West - Suite 403
Los Angeles, CA 90067
tel: 213/277-2460

Audio Visual Medical Marketing, Inc.
404 Park Avenue South
New York, NY 10016
tel: 212/532-9400

Audio Visual Narrative Arts, Inc.
Box 9
Pleasantville, NY 10570
tel: 914/769-8545

Benchmark Films, Inc.
145 Scarborough Road
Briar Cliff Manor, NY 10510
tel: 914/762-3838

Berkeley Hospice Training Project
2728 Durant Avenue
Berkeley, CA 94704
tel: 415/548-8433

Boston Family Institute
251 Harvard Street
Brookline, MA 02146
tel: 617/731-2883

Vince Books
Department of Radio-Television-Film
Annenberg Hall
Temple University
Philadelphia, PA 19122
tel: 215/787-8483

Robert J. Brady Co.
Bowie, MD 20715
tel: 301/262-6300

CRM/McGraw-Hill Films
110 15th Street
Del Mar, CA 92014
tel: 714/453-5000

Carousel (CBS) Films, Inc.
1501 Broadway
New York, NY 10036
tel: 212/354-0315

College of Pharmacy and Allied
  Health Professions
Northeastern University
306 Huntington Avenue
Boston, MA 02115

Communications in Learning, Inc.
2280 Main Street
Buffalo, NY 14214
tel: 716/837-7555

Concept Media
P.O. Box 19542
Irvine, CA 92713
tel: 714/833-3347

Concern for Dying
250 West 57th Street
New York, NY 10107
tel: 212/246-6962

Coronet/Perspective Films
65 East South Water Street
Chicago, IL 60601
tel: 312/977-4000

Council on Education and Science
Pennsylvania Medical Society
20 Erford Road
Lemoyne, PA 17043
tel: 717/763-7151

Creative Marketing
910 South 9th Street
Springfield, IL 62703
tel: 217/528-1756

Department of Physical Medicine
  and Rehabilitation
860 Mayo Building - Box 297
University of Minnesota
Minneapolis, MN 55455
tel: 612/373-9198

Embassy of the Netherlands
4200 Linnean Avenue, N.W.
Washington, DC 20008
tel: 202/244-5300

Emory Medical Television Network
Glenn Building
Emory University School of Medicine
69 Butler Street, S.E.
Atlanta, GA 30303
tel: 404/659-5307

Encyclopedia Britannica Educational
  Corporation
425 North Michigan Avenue
Department 10A
Chicago, IL 60611
tel: 312/321-6800

Edward Feil Productions
4614 Prospect Avenue
Cleveland, OH 44103
tel: 216/771-0655

Filmakers Library, Inc.
133 East 58th Street
New York, NY 10022
tel: 212/355-6545

Films, Inc.
733 Green Bay Road
Wilmette, IL 60091
tel: 800/323-4222
       312/256-3200

Great Plains National Instructional
  Television Library
P.O. Box 80669
Lincoln, NB 68501
tel: 402/472-2007

Greenhaven Press
577 Shoreview Park Road
St. Paul, MN 55112
tel: 612/482-1582

Grove Press
Film Division
196 West Houston Street
New York, NY 10014
tel: 212/242-4900

Dr. Edmund G. Howe
Department of Psychiatry
Uniformed Services University
  of the Health Sciences
School of Medicine
4301 Jones Bridge Road
Bethesda, MD 20014
tel: 202/295-3097

Indiana University
Audio-Visual Center
Bloomington, IN 47405
tel: 812/337-8087

King Features Entertainment, Inc.
235 East 45th Street
New York, NY 10017
tel: 800/223-7383
       212/682-5600

Learning Corporation of America
1350 Avenue of the Americas
New York, NY 10019
tel: 212/397-9330

Learning Resources Center
Bio-Information Center
Creighton University
28th and Burt
Omaha, NB 68178
tel: 402/280-2571

Lowengard & Brotherhood
12 Charter Oaks Place
Hartford, CT 06106
tel: 203/525-4471

MacMillan Films, Inc.
34 MacQuestern Parkway South
Mt. Vernon, NY 10550
tel: 916/664-5051

Dr. Thomas R. McCormick
c/o 4525 19th Avenue, N.E.
Seattle, WA 98109
tel: 206/524-7900

McGraw-Hill
Princeton Road
Hightstown, NJ 08520
tel: 609/448-9060

Michigan Media
416 Fourth Street
Ann Arbor, MI 48109
tel: 313/764-5360

National Audiovisual Center
National Archives and Records Service
General Services Administration
Washington, DC 20409
tel: 301/763-1896

National Film Board of Canada
1251 Avenue of the Americas
New York, NY 10020
tel: 212/586-5131

National Medical Audiovisual Center
c/o Modern Talking Pictures
  Service, Inc.
5000 Park Street
St. Petersburg, FL 33709
tel: 813/541-7571

National Public Radio
Customer Service Department
P.O. Box 216
Niles, MI 49120
tel: 800/253-0808
      616/471-3402

The Ohio Program in the Humanities
680 College Avenue
Columbus, OH 43209
tel: 614/236-6879

PBS Video
475 L'Enfant Plaza, S.W.
Washington, DC 20024
tel: 800/424-7963
      202/488-5220

Pacifica Tape Library
5316 Venice Boulevard
Los Angeles, CA 90019
tel: 213/931-1625

Pennsylvania State University
Audio Visual Services
Special Services Building
University Park, PA 16802
tel: 814/865-6314

Perennial Education, Inc.
477 Roger Williams
P.O. Box 855
Ravinia
Highland Park, IL 60035
tel: 800/323-9084
      312/433-1610

Phoenix Films, Inc.
468 Park Avenue South
New York, NY 10016
tel: 800/221-1274
      212/684-5910

Polymorph Films
118 South Street
Boston, MA 02116
tel: 617/542-2004

Professional Research
12960 Coral Tree Place
Los Angeles, CA 90066
tel: 800/421-2363
      213/823-1122

Pyramid Film and Video
Box 1048
Santa Monica, CA 90406
tel: 800/421-2304
      213/828-7577

Mrs. Esther Ruiz
Television Center, Room ES 802
Biomedical Communications
The University of Texas
Health Sciences Center at Dallas
5323 Harry Hines Boulevard
Dallas, TX 75235
tel: 214/688-3692

St. Louis University Medical Center
Audiovisual Department
1402 South Grand Avenue
St. Louis, MO 63104
tel: 314/664-9800 ext. 124

Science and Mankind, Inc.
Communications Park
Box 2000
Mt. Kisco, NY 10549
tel: 800/431-1242
      914/666-4100

Sunburst Communications
39 Washington Avenue
Pleasantville, NY 10570
tel: 800/431-1934
      914/768-5030

Time-Life Video Distribution Center
100 Eisenhower Drive
P.O. Box 644
Paramus, NJ 07652
tel: 201/843-4545

The Trainex Health Care Library
P.O. Box 116
Garden Grove, CA 92642
tel: 800/854-2485
      800/472-2479 (California
                     residents)

Dr. John S. Trumbold
Scripps Memorial Hospital
Cancer Center Films
P.O. Box 28
La Jolla, CA 92038
tel: 714/457-6756

University of Arizona
College of Medicine
Arizona Health Sciences Center
Division of Biomedical Communications
Tucson, AZ 85724
tel: 602/626-0111

University of California
  at Los Angeles
Instructional Media Library
Royce Hall, Room 8
405 Hilgard Avenue
Los Angeles, CA 90024
tel: 213/825-0755

University of Virginia
School of Medicine
The Claude Moore Health Sciences
  Library
P.O. Box 395, Medical Center
Charlottesville, VA 22908
tel: 804/924-5521

University of Washington Press
4045 Brooklyn Avenue, N.E.
Seattle, WA 98105
tel: 206/543-4050

WBGU-TV
Bowling Green State University
Bowling Green, OH 43403
tel: 419/372-0121

Dr. Robert B. White
Department of Psychiatry and
  Behavioral Sciences
University of Texas
Medical Branch at Galveston
Galveston, TX 77550
tel: 713/765-1281

Zipporah Films
54 Lewis Wharf
Boston, MA 02110
tel: 617/742-6680

This book is one of four publications intended to engage a broad range of persons in informed decision-making regarding key health and human value questions. Each publication has a usefulness of its own, while all four comprise a convenient series.

In this book, Human Values in Medicine and Health Care: Audio-Visual Resources, approximately 400 audio-visual items are listed; most are annotated, and all provide full information about purchase and rental costs and the names and addresses of distributors. Two indexes list the items by topic and by format (film, videocassette, audio-cassette, or slide/tape).

Also available in the series are:

*   Health and Human Values: A Guide to Making Your Own Decisions, by Frank Harron, John Burnside, M.D., and Tom Beauchamp. The main text contains case studies and background discussions of important moral, medical, and legal topics, selected readings from prominent writers in medicine, theology, philosophy, law, and related fields, and annotated bibliographies of recommended articles, books, anthologies, literary works, and audio-visual resources.

*   Leader's Manual for Health and Human Values: A Guide to Making Your Own Decisions. For persons leading study groups, continuing professional education courses, and academic classes concentrating on biomedical-ethical issues, this manual offers suggestions for making best use of the cases and discussions in the primary study book, organizing learning activities, and selecting further references for group discussion.

*   Biomedical-Ethical Issues: A Digest of Law and Policy Development. This handbook contains excerpts and summaries of influential court decisions, state and federal legislation, and federal guidelines, as well as policy statements from various religious and professional organizations, related to biomedical-ethical issues. By providing excerpts, the digest enables the general reader and the legal specialist to understand the recent evolution of public policy and to recognize those areas of public policy that remain incomplete and, in some cases, contradictory.

These publications are offered to the general reader, patients and their families, physicians, nurses, and other health care practitioners, clergy, attorneys, educators, students, legislators, and activists who seek to influence public policy. It is hoped that they will be used to help inform our thinking about the crucial health and human value choices facing us all today.

Ordering Information

To place an order for any book in the Health and Human Values series, write or call: Yale University Press, Sales Department, 92A Yale Station, New Haven, CT 06520; Tel. (203) 432-4840.